Small Animal Euthanasia: Updates on Clinical Practice

Editors

BETH MARCHITELLI
TAMARA SHEARER

VETERINARY CLINICS OF NORTH AMERICA: SMALL ANIMAL PRACTICE

www.vetsmall.theclinics.com

May 2020 • Volume 50 • Number 3

ELSEVIER

1600 John F. Kennedy Boulevard • Suite 1800 • Philadelphia, Pennsylvania, 19103-2899

http://www.vetsmall.theclinics.com

VETERINARY CLINICS OF NORTH AMERICA: SMALL ANIMAL PRACTICE Volume 50, Number 3
May 2020 ISSN 0195-5616, ISBN-13: 978-0-323-72076-2

Editor: Colleen Dietzler
Developmental Editor: Nicole Congleton

Veterinary Clinics of North America: Small Animal Practice (ISSN 0195-5616) is published bimonthly by Elsevier Inc., 360 Park Avenue South, New York, NY 10010-1710. Months of issue are January, March, May, July, September, and November. Business and Editorial Offices: 1600 John F. Kennedy Blvd., Ste. 1800, Philadelphia, PA 19103-2899. Customer Service Office: 3251 Riverport Lane, Maryland Heights, MO 63043. Periodicals postage paid at New York, NY and additional mailing offices. Subscription prices are $348.00 per year (domestic individuals), $705.00 per year (domestic institutions), $100.00 per year (domestic students/residents), $451.00 per year (Canadian individuals), $876.00 per year (Canadian institutions), $488.00 per year (international individuals), $876.00 per year (international institutions), $100.00 per year (Canadian students/residents), and $220.00 per year (international students/residents). To receive student/resident rate, orders must be accompanied by name of affiliated institution, date of term, and the *signature* of program/residency coordinator on institution letterhead. Orders will be billed at individual rate until proof of status is received. Foreign air speed delivery is included in all *Clinics* subscription prices. All prices are subject to change without notice. **POSTMASTER:** Send address changes to *Veterinary Clinics of North America: Small Animal Practice*, Elsevier Health Sciences Division, Subscription Customer Service, 3251 Riverport Lane, Maryland Heights, MO 63043. Customer Service (orders, claims, online, change of address): Elsevier Periodicals Customer Service, Elsevier Health Sciences Division Subscription **Customer Service 3251 Riverport Lane Maryland Heights, MO 63043. Tel: 1-800-654-2452 (U.S. and Canada); 314-447-8871 (outside U.S. and Canada). Fax: 314-447-8029. E-mail: journalscustomerservice-usa@elsevier.com (for print support); journalsonlinesupport-usa@elsevier.com (for online support).**

Reprints. For copies of 100 or more of articles in this publication, please contact the Commercial Reprints Department, Elsevier Inc., 360 Park Avenue South, New York, NY 10010-1710. Tel.: 212-633-3874; Fax: 212-633-3820; E-mail: reprints@elsevier.com.

Veterinary Clinics of North America: Small Animal Practice is also published in Japanese by Inter Zoo Publishing Co., Ltd., Aoyama Crystal-Bldg 5F, 3-5-12 Kitaaoyama, Minato-ku, Tokyo 107-0061, Japan.

Veterinary Clinics of North America: Small Animal Practice is covered in *Current Contents/Agriculture, Biology and Environmental Sciences, Science Citation Index, ASCA, MEDLINE/PubMed (Index Medicus), Excerpta Medica, and BIOSIS.*

Contributors

EDITORS

BETH MARCHITELLI, DVM, MS
Founder/Owner, 4 Paws Farewell: Mobile Pet Hospice, Palliative Care and Home
Euthanasia, Asheville, North Carolina

TAMARA SHEARER, DVM, MS, CCRP, CVPP, CVA, CHPV, CTPEP
Founder/Owner, Smoky Mountain Integrative Veterinary Clinic, Sylva, North Carolina;
Faculty, Chi Institute, Reddick, Florida

AUTHORS

MARK D. CARLSON, DVM
Stow Kent Animal Hospital, Kent, Ohio

KELLY CARTER, RVT
4 Paws Farewell: Mobile Pet Hospice, Palliative Care and Home Euthanasia, Asheville,
North Carolina

NATHANIEL COOK, DVM, CVA, CVFT, CTPEP
Chicago Veterinary Geriatrics, Chicago, Illinois

KATHLEEN COONEY, DVM, MS, CHPV, CCFP
Founder and Director, Education, Companion Animal Euthanasia Training Academy
(CAETA), Loveland, Colorado

MARY GARDNER, DVM
Lap of Love, Boynton Beach, Florida

MARY LUMMIS, DVM
4 Paws Farewell: Mobile Pet Hospice, Palliative Care and Home Euthanasia, Asheville,
North Carolina

BETH MARCHITELLI, DVM, MS
Founder/Owner, 4 Paws Farewell: Mobile Pet Hospice, Palliative Care and Home
Euthanasia, Asheville, North Carolina

ROBERT E. MEYER, DVM
Diplomate, American College of Veterinary Anesthesia and Analgesia; Board Certified
Specialist in Veterinary Anesthesia and Analgesia, Professor, Veterinary Anesthesiology,
College of Veterinary Medicine, Mississippi State, Mississippi

LAUREN ORVIN, DVM, CHPV
Lowcountry Pet Hospice and Home Euthanasia, Moncks Corner, South Carolina

JESSICA PIERCE, PhD
Faculty Affiliate, Center for Bioethics and Humanities, University of Colorado Anschutz
Medical Campus, Aurora, Colorado

SHEILAH A. ROBERTSON, BVMS (Hons), PhD, MRCVS
Diplomate of the American College of Veterinary Anesthesia and Analgesia; Diplomate of the European College of Anaesthesia and Analgesia; Diplomate of the American College of Animal Welfare; Diplomate of the European College of Animal Welfare and Behavioural Medicine (Welfare, Science, Ethics and Law), Lap of Love Veterinary Hospice Inc., Lutz, Florida

TAMARA SHEARER, DVM, MS, CCRP, CVPP, CVA, CHPV, CTPEP
Founder/Owner, Smoky Mountain Integrative Veterinary Clinic, Sylva, North Carolina; Faculty, Chi Institute, Reddick, Florida

MARY BETH SPITZNAGEL, PhD
Associate Professor, Department of Psychological Sciences, Kent State University, Kent Hall, Kent, Ohio

Contents

The history of companion animal euthanasia includes a blend of good and bad methodology, the shifting landscape of the human-animal bond, and maturation of the veterinary euthanasia experience. Time has shown us that critical exploration of what once was acceptable will lead the way to modern best practices. Animal welfare remains at the heart of the procedure, with equally matched attention now given to client and veterinary team well-being. Although euthanasia will continue to evolve, it is clear through the twenty-first century advancements, a tipping point of necessary change is upon us.

The science of transitional states of consciousness is reviewed. Despite intensive study, determining the subjective experience of animals during transitional states of consciousness remains inherently limited. Until better assessment tools become available, behavior-based observations, such as loss of righting reflex/loss of posture, remain among our most useful guides to the onset of unconsciousness in animals. To minimize potential animal suffering and to ensure a truly unconscious state is unambiguously achieved, a state of general anesthesia relying on gamma amino butyric acid type A agonists or N-methyl-d-aspartate antagonist agents continues to be a necessary component of the companion animal euthanasia process.

The pathophysiology of dying and death, related to veterinary patients, has warranted less attention than normal and abnormal physiologic processes related to life preservation. In addition, many veterinary patients are euthanized, which prevents observation of natural disease progression, while ameliorating suffering. Acute death in human medicine can serve as a model for understanding mechanisms of death in veterinary patients under certain conditions. The specific cause of cardiac arrest in several different models of disease elucidates end-stage disease processes. Understanding the path to death and dying in veterinary patients physiologically serves to guide best practices focused on alleviating suffering.

Video content accompanies this article at http://www.vetsmall. theclinics.com

Pre-euthanasia sedation or anesthesia offers many benefits. It allows the owners to spend time with their pet before euthanasia, improves safety for the person performing euthanasia and others who are present, decreases stress for the patient, reduces or eliminates the need for physical restraint for intravenous injection. Under anesthesia, non-intravenous routes may be used for administration of euthanasia solutions. Some drugs that do not require injection; the oral transmucosal route is noninvasive and suitable for several drugs or drug combinations. The oral route also is feasible, but there are fewer data available on suitable drugs and doses.

There are many acceptable routes of euthanasia solution administration in companion animals. The most common ones are those with consistent use and success, and that align with what is best for the patient, client, and veterinary team. Common injection sites include the venous, hepatic, and renal systems. The barbiturate drugs are in consistent use today, but other drugs may be better given the setting and circumstances at the time. Alternative techniques are available, but only reached for when other more suitable routes of administration are not ideal.

Data collection and research about adverse effects associated with euthanasia are lacking in the veterinary profession. The goal of this article is to review current research about euthanasia and propose concepts to collect and document euthanasia data to support future studies. A better understanding of the side effects witnessed near perimortem should provide benefits to pet owners, veterinarians, and staff, especially if methods are uncovered to minimize or mitigate the adverse events witnessed. Such data can provide valuable insight and guidance in improving the quality of death and furthering education about the dying process.

This article reviews factors contributing to the decision to euthanize a patient by exploring the diagnosis, clinical signs, and triggers behind the choice. By investigating these triggers, the article helps guide practitioners to proactively manage areas of concern that lead to the decision of euthanasia. Included in this article is a benchmark comprehensive survey for pet families that standardizes documentation of family decision making surrounding end of life and euthanasia. Increased knowledge about diagnosis, clinical signs, and triggers may improve the technical and communication skills of professionals about specific conditions that are encountered at the end of life.

Euthanasia from the Veterinary Client's Perspective: Psychosocial Contributors to Euthanasia Decision Making

Mary Beth Spitznagel, Beth Marchitelli, Mary Gardner, and Mark D. Carlson

End-of-life decision making for a companion animal relies on the veterinarian acting as educator and counselor. However, little research has been conducted to understand client variables in this context. The current study examined potential client-related contributors to steps taken toward a euthanasia decision. Caregiver burden, anticipatory grief, depression, stress, and income all correlated positively with this outcome. However, when client factors were examined in a regression model controlling for animal quality of life, only caregiver burden and income emerged as significant predictors. All 3 caregiver burden factors: general strain, affective/relational discomfort, and guilt/uncertainty were significantly related to consideration of euthanasia.

Communication: Difficult Conversation In Veterinary End-of-Life Care

Mary Lummis, Beth Marchitelli, and Tamara Shearer

 Video content accompanies this article at http://www.vetsmall. theclinics.com.

This article demonstrates how good communication sets the foundation to provide superior comprehensive care during the stressful time surrounding end of life. Communication addressing end-of-life care in veterinary medicine has significant impact on all involved: the patient, the client, the health care team, and the practice. These conversations require training and practice to achieve mutually satisfying outcomes. Suggested guides for facilitating these conversations and several typical scenarios are presented to provide methods for future evidenced-based evaluation in effective communication. The Critical Incident Stress Management is presented as a model for mitigation of adverse consequences related to traumatic events in veterinary practice.

A Comparison of Human and Animal Assisted Dying Protocols

Beth Marchitelli and Jessica Pierce

This article compares human and veterinary assisted dying protocols, exploring the relevant similarities and differences in the practice of euthanasia between these related fields of medicine. Special focus is placed on the use of medical terminology and technical application of drug protocols. Comparative research in this area may provide useful insights for the fields of veterinary medicine and human medicine alike.

VETERINARY CLINICS OF NORTH AMERICA: SMALL ANIMAL PRACTICE

SERIES OF RELATED INTEREST

Veterinary Clinics of North America: Exotic Animal Practice
https://www.vetexotic.theclinics.com/

THE CLINICS ARE NOW AVAILABLE ONLINE!
Access your subscription at:
www.theclinics.com

Preface

Small Animal Euthanasia: Future Practice and Clinical Application

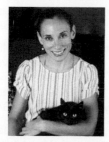   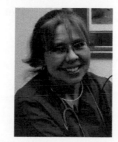

Beth Marchitelli, DVM, MS   Tamara Shearer, DVM, MS
Editors

We are delighted to have participated in the publication of this issue of *Veterinary Clinics of North America: Small Animal Practice* on Euthanasia: Updates on Clinical Practice. This issue is unique in that it is the first of its kind to focus exclusively on the clinical practice of companion animal euthanasia. Increased demand for services focused exclusively on hospice, palliative care, and home euthanasia for companion animals has brought scrutiny to the technical and procedural aspects of small animal euthanasia. Empirical evidence in this context, although sparse, is emerging to guide best practices. The weight of emotional burden coupled with the ethical and moral responsibility practitioners and pet owners face when euthanizing family pets warrants interdisciplinary evaluation and scientific support. The study of small animal euthanasia requires attention from various disciplines. Such a comprehensive approach ensures that the profession devotes the appropriate relevancy and importance the practice of euthanasia requires in everyday clinical practice. This issue evaluates small animal euthanasia from varying perspectives: clinical and technical application and social and psychological impact on the family as caregiver. It also pushes the boundaries of scientific understanding regarding transitional states of consciousness and new areas of study relevant to euthanasia decision making. We intentionally did not include sections on the impact of the practice of euthanasia on veterinary practitioners in the form of compassion fatigue and burnout nor did we address the affects of pet loss and bereavement on caregivers. In addition, we excluded euthanasia techniques and practices for small mammals, birds, and exotics. Although these are worthy topics, we opted to exclude them because of extensive existing professional and academic literature on these topics. This issue seeks to explore areas that have previously been overlooked, such as comparison to the terminology and practice of medical aid in dying in human medicine and our current understanding of brain states in the context of euthanasia. We hope this issue proves fascinating in its own right and at the same time is relevant to everyday practice.

Special thanks are extended to Kelly Carter, Heather Carter, Beth Rhyne, Becky Rhoades, Mary Lummis, Amy Pruitt, Patricia Robertson, Caren Harris, Mary Jo Bale, and Mike Mericer.

Beth Marchitelli, DVM, MS
4 Paws Farewell: Mobile Pet Hospice
Palliative Care and Home Euthanasia
Asheville, NC, USA

Tamara Shearer, DVM, MS
Smoky Mountain Integrative
Veterinary Clinic
1054 Haywood Road
Sylva, NC 28779, USA

E-mail addresses:
bmarchitelli@hotmail.com (B. Marchitelli)
tshearer5@frontier.com (T. Shearer)

Historical Perspective of Euthanasia in Veterinary Medicine

Kathleen Cooney, DVM, MS, CHPV, CCFP

KEYWORDS

• Euthanasia • Death • Dysthanasia • Hospice • Pentobarbital • Education • Mobile

KEY POINTS

- There is a blend of good and bad methods throughout the history of companion animal euthanasia.
- The well-being of the animal as well as the client and veterinary team are important in modern practices.
- The euthanasia process will continue to evolve as twenty-first century advancements continue to emerge.

INTRODUCTION

Writing an article on the history of small animal euthanasia has proven a very hefty endeavor. There is a profound amount of information to consider including. What has been laid out is the blueprint of where we have come from and how we have arrived at our present ideas of what constitutes a good death today. Much of what is written here comes from early versions of the American Veterinary Medical Association (AVMA)'s euthanasia guidelines, the Massachusetts Society for the Prevention of Cruelty to Animals (SPCA) archives, ethics and philosophy books, the American Veterinary Medical History Society, and my own personal communication with leaders in the field. The following is a blend of objective and subjective material taken with only a hint of the necessary context needed to fully appreciate the culture of the day. My hope is to get the reader thinking about the legacy of the past and mood of today as the chaperon to our future.

To help set the stage of this article, and the reverent tone of the issue itself, it is worthwhile to share some viewpoints of noted writers who helped shape the perception of euthanasia in veterinary medicine.

- Taken from *Euthanasia of the Companion Animal*, Paul Langner[1]
  "Here is respect for the nature of the animal, recognition of its individuality and

Education, Companion Animal Euthanasia Training Academy (CAETA), Loveland, CO, USA
E-mail address: cooneydvm@gmail.com

Vet Clin Small Anim 50 (2020) 489–502
https://doi.org/10.1016/j.cvsm.2019.12.001
0195-5616/20/© 2019 Elsevier Inc. All rights reserved.

intrinsic worth, concern over achieving a rapid, unstressful, and dignified death, and a sense of relief when this goal is successfully reached."
- Taken from *Animal Rights and Human Morality*, Bernie Rollin[2]
  "To be forced to kill something you love in order to ensure that it not suffer is an awesome burden. Those of us who have been forced to have an animal euthanized because it was suffering know that this experience is one that one never forgets."
- Taken from *Blue Juice*, Patricia Morris[3]
  "You can tell a lot about a veterinarian by the way he or she handles euthanasia. How you end your patient's life can be just as important as healing the patient."
- Taken from *The Last Walk*, Jessica Pierce[4]
  "It would be nice to live in a world where "dying like an animal" signified a peaceful, respectful, and meaningful death."

NAMING EUTHANASIA

The term euthanasia has gone through an evolution since its origin in 121 AD. Derived from Greek, euthanasia is the combination of the root words, "Eu," meaning good, and "Thanatos," meaning death. The first recorded use of the word is attributed to the Roman historian, Suetonius, in his book, *The Lives of the Caesars*, and how, in particular, their goal when death drew near was to achieve "euthanasia" or gentle death. He used the term euthanasia to signify an easy death, a death not associated with the act of taking life, but rather just experiencing the quintessential gentle end: loved ones gathered close, peace and acceptance that death has come, and all affairs in order. Suetonius describes how the emperor Augustus, dying quickly and without suffering, in the arms of his wife, experienced the "euthanasia" he had hoped for.[5] In the 1600s, the noted scientist, philosopher, and advisor to the Queen of England, Sir Francis Bacon, used the term euthanasia again in much the same way in an effort to try to convince the medical community to pay attention to the dying, to do more for those suffering death.[6] He was frustrated with the medical community for leaving patients to suffer unnecessarily. Bacon wanted medical advancements to alleviate pain and suffering so the dying could achieve their desired euthanasia. What is interesting to me is that Bacon, along with many others I am sure, was ultimately seeking palliative medicine, a field of study that would remain largely unavailable until the invention of more modern medicine some 300 years later. For both Suetonius and Bacon, euthanasia was a passive, descriptive term.

In 1870, the definition of euthanasia changed forever through the published work of a British schoolteacher named Samuel Williams. A supporter of the eugenics (from the Greek "eu", good, and "genos", race) movement of the time, Williams published a literary paper using the term "euthanasia" meaning to actively take life. He proposed that actively ending life was a generosity to the dying and to society as a whole.[6] By administering a toxin, it was possible to forego unnecessary lingering and subsequent risk of spreading disease or other infallibility that would bring danger to the human populous. His message grew in popularity and eventually led to the acceptable practice of euthanasia as we know it today. Although not commonly practiced in human medicine until more recently, the use of active euthanasia in animal science and veterinary medicine has been around for hundreds of years, even though it may have been termed something different, like mercy killing or necessary death to eliminate suffering. The manner in which animal death is carried out has transformed from only physical methods to include more advanced use of targeted drugs and chemicals.

The term euthanasia is used today to describe death from a variety of angles, such as mercy killing of the sick and suffering, to shelter depopulation. It is a catchall for all manner of death, a point that the AVMA recognized in their 2013 guidelines.[7] After talking with several ethicists and sociologists, it seemed no one was interested in taking on the daunting task of creating new nomenclature. Within veterinary medicine, euthanasia remains a word used for the procedure or act of taking life to eliminate suffering, with minimal to no suffering by the animal in question (see Beth Marchitelli and Jessica Pierce's article, "A Comparison of Human and Animal Assisted Dying Protocols," in this issue). We will see if other terms arise that better define ending life for alternative purposes. The word dysthanasia was proposed as a suitable antonym to euthanasia in 2017.[8] By giving a distinct word to a bad death experience, the objective is to enhance a veterinary team's ability to target and address the negative situation. When a dysthanasia occurs and is labeled as such, a clear plan of resolution can be set in motion, that is, client communication, altering protocols based on similar patient parameters, team debriefing, and so forth.

Euphemisms to soften the reality of euthanasia have gained in popularity, I speculate in conjunction with the growth of the human-animal bond. A euphemism is a mild or indirect word or expression substituted for one considered to be too harsh when referring to something unpleasant.[9] Because of the emotional nature of euthanasia and the fact that it can be difficult to explain to children or those who would have a difficult time understanding the reality of death, euphemisms soften the cold hard facts. However, we also know euphemisms can lead to confusion and can do more harm than good. The terms that have developed over time include "put to sleep," "put down," and "cross over the Rainbow Bridge." To describe the death itself, you may have heard "passed away" or simply "he's gone."

Active Versus Passive

There are 2 adjectives classically used when describing euthanasia: active and passive. The following definitions were taken from the book, *Euthanasia—Ethical and human aspects, Volume One*, published by the Council of Europe[10] (**Box 1**).

By my estimation, passive euthanasia is far more frequent in companion animals than is discussed. Although the slow death of a pet patient may not be the objective for most clients and veterinary teams, it nonetheless occurs when active euthanasia is

---

Box 1
Active versus passive euthanasia

1. Active (or direct) euthanasia signifies the act of causing death deliberately by administering a toxic substance or acute physical method leading to death, ideally within a few minutes. (When we consider the classic manifestation of euthanasia with companion animals, this is the definition that most closely reflects contemporary veterinary practices.)

2. Passive (or indirect) euthanasia means we may not be doing anything specific to end life abruptly, but rather altering a being's existence to gently bring about the end of life. There are 3 interpretations of passive euthanasia:
   - The first interpretation is the suspension of all essential treatments with the intention of ending suffering. (This is designed to reduce lingering on the verge of death. Examples are withholding food, water, oxygen.)
   - The second interpretation is suspending or rejecting all "unreasonable" treatments. (Examples are chemotherapy and artificial respiration. Although these treatments have a commanding presence in veterinary curative and palliative therapies, their absence will hasten the dying process.)
   - The third interpretation is death resulting from a necessary escalation in the dosing of sedatives administered to combat pain and/or anxiety. (This is referred to in human and animal hospice as palliative sedation, which can be increased to a forced state of unconsciousness known as continuous palliative sedation.)[11]

not chosen and life-sustaining therapies are avoided. The culture of open and honest communication, including client education around matters of death, has been moving in the right direction. Veterinary teams are better equipped today to guide clients around when or when not to choose euthanasia and to address client concerns regarding its necessity and ethical decision making than even 10 years ago.

THE AMERICAN VETERINARY MEDICAL ASSOCIATION GUIDELINES AND HISTORICAL METHODS

The evolution of modern medicine has provided safer and more humane methods of euthanasia. There was no doubt many felt concern and disdain over earlier forms of killing. To watch an animal struggle with death forces one to reflect on one's own morality. It is hard and unsettling to watch another being gasp for air, writhe in pain, and/ or vocalize in agony. It is an unsustainable ordeal that forced necessary change in our euthanasia methods throughout much of the twentieth century. The first big push for organized veterinary medicine euthanasia reform came in the early 1960s. The AVMA, at the request of the Council on Research, gathered together the top minds in veterinary medicine and welfare to write methodology and guidelines. The first published Report of the AVMA Panel on Euthanasia came in 1963. Listing only 7 criteria for method selection, the report focused heavily on methods and techniques. All known methods in use at the time were included, with emphasis on advantages and disadvantages of each, plus recommendations on how to work with certain species while maintaining personnel safety. What I so appreciate about the early reports is the firm stance taken on some techniques as unacceptable under any circumstance, such as with the use of strychnine and hydrocyanic acid, especially at a time when the use of preeuthanasia sedation or anesthesia was rare.

As the years and revisions went on, increased attention was given to behavioral considerations, pain perception, species considerations, witness experience, and available research. Also included were clear distinctions around which methods/techniques were Acceptable, Acceptable with Conditions, Unacceptable, and which methods were to be used as adjuncts to others.[7] In 2013, the Report was retitled AVMA Guidelines for the Euthanasia of Animals. Panel member size also expanded to aid in addressing the complexities of the available methods and ethical discussion. With respect to all that has been written within the Reports and Guidelines, it is important to distinguish the Guidelines are just that, guidelines. They are not law per se and speak to the importance of one's expert opinion guiding technique choice given each case's unique situation. In other words, it is up to the one performing euthanasia to make the best decisions based on the known information. The veterinary team is to follow the scientific and empirical recommendations of the experts and blend it compassionately for the benefit of the patient in front of them. Should one ignore these recommendations, a malpractice claim is possible, and likely, depending on how severely the pet in question suffered at their hand.

Euthanasia may be performed by licensed veterinarians, licensed veterinary technicians (in some US states), shelter euthanasia technicians, law enforcement, and even laypersons when the animal poses severe danger to the public at large.[11] Licensed veterinarians are able to obtain the necessary controlled drugs for injections and monitor their use by others in their jurisdiction. In the hospital setting, veterinarians remain the director of care and ultimate authority on euthanasia approval.

The euthanasia methods used in veterinary medicine are rooted in 14 criteria aimed to ensure death is permanent, pain and suffering (by all involved) are minimized, and safety is attained. Other groups, like the Institute for the Study of Animal Problems, in a report dated August 1978, followed similar criteria[7] (**Box 2**).

Box 2
The 14 criteria for euthanasia method evaluation
1. Ability to induce loss of consciousness and death with minimal pain or anxiety
2. Time to induce unconsciousness
3. Reliability
4. Safety of personnel
5. Irreversibility
6. Compatibility with requirement and purpose
7. Emotional effect on observers/operators
8. Compatibility with subsequent evaluation/examination/use of tissue
9. Drug availability and human abuse potential
10. Compatibility with species, age, health status
11. Ability to maintain equipment in proper working order
12. Legal requirements
13. Safety for predators/scavengers
14. Environmental impacts from both methods and animal remains
Data from American Veterinary Medical Association. AVMA Guidelines for the Euthanasia of Animals: 2013 Edition. Schaumburg, IL: American Veterinary Medical Association; 2013. Available at: https://www.avma.org/sites/default/files/resources/euthanasia.pdf.

Methods: the Good and not so Good

Since the beginning of recorded euthanasia methodology, veterinary medicine has grouped methods into 3 main categories of delivery: noninhalant pharmaceutical administration, inhalant gases, and physical methods. The goal of each is to render the animal unconscious as quickly as possible, followed by cessation of life either immediately or within a short period of time. Each method consists of a variety of means/agents, all with pros and cons. Most of the time, veterinary professionals settle in on one they like best and can routinely rely on. In small animal clinical practice, this would be the noninhalant pharmaceuticals, followed by inhalant gases, then last and certainly least, the physical methods. Using a captive bolt or gunshot for an old cat is a far cry from ideal and reserved only for extreme situations when nothing else will do, especially when clients are present.

When available, inhalant gases were used to induce death. In the heyday of ether and chloroform, these gases were regularly given to puppies and kittens. Adult animals were not sensitive enough to it and had prolonged death times. Other gases included hydrogen cyanide, carbon dioxide, and carbon monoxide. Carbon monoxide was administered in chambers or in the backs of trucks. There are numerous accounts of using truck exhaust as a means to deliver carbon monoxide gas to animals in animal control vehicles (although not necessarily common practice in veterinary hospitals, it is nevertheless part of our history). Instructions were written out how best to accomplish this, with data showing it was most effective when the truck was idling. Carbon dioxide is another gas delivered in chambers, but was challenging because of the high volume of gas required. Pets also found it aversive to breathe (air hunger), and descriptions report live animals climbing on top of dead ones to find oxygen up high. In situations whereby injectable agents were unavailable, veterinarians had to resort to whatever method was quick, affordable, and thought to be humane at the time.

Noninhalant drug administration is our main form of euthanasia in traditional veterinary hospitals and really has been since the discovery and availability of barbiturates. It is interesting to note when reading through old versions of the AVMA's Euthanasia Guidelines how drugs were given to pets in many of the same ways we do today, but without the benefit of preeuthanasia sedation or anesthesia. There are some early reports of their benefit, but it was not considered common practice. Routes of injectable drug administration included intravenous, intracardiac, intraperitoneal, intrathecal, intrathoracic, intramuscular, subcutaneous, orally, and rectally. The first AVMA euthanasia guidelines talked about intracardiac injections on animals that were awake and how they may show signs of distress. Barbiturates, the category of drug we use most commonly today, were the clear frontrunner in superior euthanasia experiences, for both the pet and witnesses. Advantages far outweighed the disadvantages; disadvantages listed only the need for restraint and increased cost during mass depopulation. Nondesirable injectable agents included chloral hydrate, magnesium sulfate, strychnine, hydrocyanic acid, and the curariform drugs. Over time, concerned leaders removed those deemed unacceptable or made it mandatory for the pet to be rendered insensible/unconscious before such drugs could be given.

Pentobarbital Takes the Lead

Barbiturates rapidly became the leading noninhalant, as mentioned in the 1963 version of the AVMA Euthanasia Guidelines. Deemed the gentlest of the "poisons," barbiturate overdoses lead to rapid unconsciousness, cessation of breathing, and cardiac arrest. Unconsciousness before cardiac arrest was a guarantee so veterinarians could be certain awareness of death was nonexistent for the dying animal. This class of drug met all of the 14 criteria of method selection, save for a few, and even then, proper storage of barbiturates and disposal of the body was all it took to keep them on the top of the pack. Pure barbiturates held human abuse potential, and in 1972, were raised from a category III to a category II controlled drug. In an effort to reduce this abuse potential, synergistic drugs were added in to increase safety and reduce some brands back down to category IIIs. The best example of this is phenytoin sodium, a cardiotoxic substance.

Pentobarbital was originally only available in powder form. Hospitals had to mix it precisely with the right type of water, alcohol, or other diluents and often found it unstable or having the wrong pH. In the early 1980s, North American Pharmacal, now Vortech Pharmaceuticals, found the right packaging and preservative formula that allowed room temperature water to be added to the powder for easy storage and administration. Eventually, pentobarbital could be purchased in liquid form, making handling even easier. For those curious about the discovery of barbiturates, their origin can be traced back to Germany in 1864. Ludwig von Baeyer, the founding father of the Bayer Company, synthesized urea with malonic acid to create barbituric acid, later transformed by Josef von Mering and Emil Fisher into the barbiturate compound we know today. Given the earlier name Veronal, it was a drug used for insomnia and other anxiety disorders.[12] Eventually, it found its way into veterinary medicine as an anesthetic drug, that when overdosed, let to a swift and peaceful death.

THE CHANGING TIDE OF THE HOSPITAL EUTHANASIA EXPERIENCE

The euthanasia appointment has long been a staple in veterinary hospitals. It is considered one of the most common procedures carried out in all of veterinary medicine. Depending on the size of the hospital and number of patients on record, the volume of euthanasia appointments ranges from zero to 100+ per week. Hospital cultures designed to exceed community expectations with euthanasia work are inclined to market themselves as such, encouraging pet owners to choose them when the time comes, and rightfully so because they have adapted their facility to be warm and welcoming for death events. Other hospitals may be the exact opposite and avoid euthanasias whenever possible. It takes some effort to quiet the space, make preparations, and bring the team into the proper mindset for euthanasia (see Tamara Shearer's article, "Non-pharmacological Methods to Improve the Euthanasia Experience," in this issue). Regardless of the culture, all veterinary teams agree that euthanasia can be expected on any given day.

The manner in which euthanasia is carried out depends heavily on the abilities of said hospital. It is difficult to say how many today are practicing with modern standards compared with older, out-of-date ones. For example, it is now recommended to keep the client and pet together throughout the entire appointment to reduce anxiety for both. Clients are never forced to stay, but they are encouraged to remain present for every step of the process if that is their wish. In years past, it was commonplace to separate client from pet to place indwelling catheters in the treatment area, or "in the back," because of concerns of the client witnessing it.[13] Today, best practices tell us to keep the bonded pair together or at least offer the option to clients. Newer standards, outlined in **Box 3**, have gained support from groups like the AVMA, the American Animal Hospital Association (AAHA), the Fear Free program, the Companion Animal Euthanasia Training Academy (CAETA), and more as the go-to for a gentler experience.

Preplanning has taken center stage in bond-centered hospitals for quite some time. Preplanning around all the factors that make up "who, what, when, where, and how" has proven important as the ceremonial manner of the appointment has increased. In the earlier days of hospital euthanasia, asking a client, "Would you like to have a chaplain present?," may have seemed bizarre compared with today, when having a chaplain onsite is a very real option (some chaplains have devoted their entire careers to the spiritual support of pet owners). Euthanasia appointments are as close to a funeral as some clients will have for their pets, and preplanning the special touches ensures there are no regrets during a time of no do-overs.

Examination rooms perfectly suited for efficient medical examinations have not historically been well suited for meaningful euthanasias. "Comfort rooms" started gaining traction in the 1990s during the design phase of new hospitals. Architects were

---

Box 3
Examples of modern standards

Preplanning with clients in advance of the appointment

Clients allowed to be present for all manner of euthanasia techniques

Longer appointment time, often 60 minutes or more

Private entrance and exit

Other animals welcome

Preeuthanasia sedation or anesthesia provided for every pet

Intraorgan routes acceptance equal to intravenous administration

Comfort room usage

Memorialization offered

Grief support provided

requested to add in a room that could be a home away from home for both client and pet. Prebuilt hospitals wanting to follow suit had to find space or convert a traditional examination room into one with soft lighting, floor padding, and reduced outside sounds. Biophilic elements such as greenery and images of nature also became more common in the 1990s. Such space helped the pet, client, and veterinary team relax and allowed the rest of the world to fade away, if only for a bit (**Figs. 1** and **2**).

The utilization of social workers in veterinary medicine has been on the increase since the late 1970s. The University of Pennsylvania (1979; Jamie Quackenbush) and the Animal Medical Center of New York (1982; Susan Cohen) were the first hospitals on record to employ a social worker for client and staff support. Through their compassionate leadership, social workers increased veterinary team confidence by demonstrating gentle client communication and care. Today, larger specialty hospitals employ veterinary social workers to aid in managing challenging cases, pet loss, and team wellness. They, and other client-focused personnel, have added in supportive features like art therapy, grief support literature, memorial gardens, honoring ceremonies, memorial funds, and pet loss support groups.

The AVMA's PLIT (Professional Liability Insurance Trust) reports few but still significant malpractice claims of dysthanasia (bad euthanasia procedures). According to a recent conversation, notable reasons for claims include the wrong pet being euthanized, evidence of pain like vocalization, and patients biting owners before the final injection. Bites to owners appear most commonly when pets are only mildly sedated during preeuthanasia sedation, when the pet was confused and reacting negatively to stimulation. With the exception of the horrible "wrong pet being euthanized"

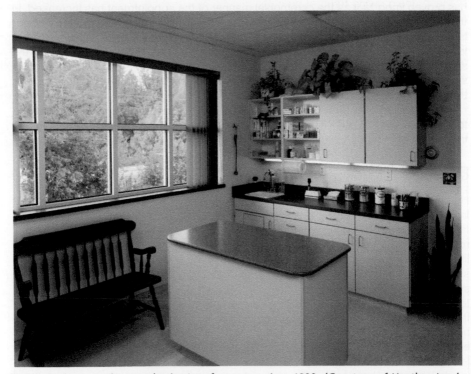

Fig. 1. Early example consultation/comfort room circa 1990. (*Courtesy of* Heather Lewis, Boulder, CO.)

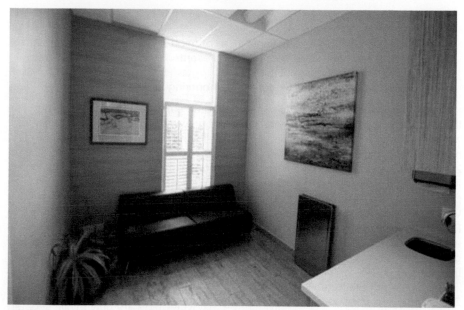

Fig. 2. Comfort room circa 2019. (*Courtesy of* Melissa Callbeck, DVM, Whitby, Ontario, Canada.)

scenario, the growing trend of preeuthanasia deep sedation or anesthesia is proving advantageous. Sleeping pets are unable to bite or vocalize during the euthanasia injection. Hospitals practicing this way find it necessary to lengthen appointment times to accommodate the sedation period and keep someone with the client and pet from beginning to end. The concept of a euthanasia attendant is newer in modern standards. Their role is to remain with the client from beginning to end, manage all expectations, and aid the veterinarian, if the veterinarian himself or herself is not the attendant. Euthanasia attendants are usually veterinary technicians/nurses or assistants well trained to handle anything that comes up, and I hope, ensure the wrong pet never gets euthanized.

GROWTH OF THE MOBILE EUTHANASIA MOVEMENT

Home euthanasia has been around since the dawn of veterinary medicine. Before the increase of brick and mortar hospitals, all veterinary medicine was carried out on the farm or in the home setting. It was normal for the animal patient to be in familiar surroundings, with other companions, and reduced handling during the last moments of life. This inherent comfort is in large part why it has regained traction today. With the shift of veterinary medicine into the hospital setting, those dedicated to the home setting share how they wish euthanasia was left out of the great medical migration, that it should have remained "back on the farm." Without being able to fully appreciate the ramifications of the hospital environment (and let us consider hospitals were not nearly as busy back then as they are today), who can blame the logic of bringing euthanasia along. I imagine many twentieth century veterinarians always preferred offering home services, regardless of how well they could offer hospital comfort, and would leave their hospitals for hours at a time to provide it.

Home euthanasia is considered especially beneficial for the following reasons:

- Comfortable setting
- Privacy
- No driving required in an emotional state of mind
- Other pets and family members can be present
- Added simplicity for home burial
- Increased time and space for ceremony/honoring services

Since around the year 2000, the number of home euthanasia services has been on the steady increase. In 2009, the online directory, www.inhomepeteuthanasia.com, was created as a resource to provide the pet-loving community the means to find home-centric veterinary teams. The directory administrator reports that as of 2019, more than 600 services have been listed or are currently listed, to help families find assistance with mobile euthanasia. Other Web sites dedicated to pet loss support host similar lists. Veterinarian-owned companies, most notably Lap of Love Veterinary Hospice and In-home Euthanasia, and Pet Loss at Home, In Home Pet Euthanasia, are multilocation mobile services with doctors serving families in cities across the United States. These and other mobile veterinarians show marked growth in requests for home euthanasia for dogs, cats, exotics, and companion livestock.

The signing of the Veterinary Medicine Mobility Act (HR 1528) into law August 1, 2014 made the transport of controlled substances into the field much easier for home euthanasia services. Up until this time, the Drug Enforcement Agency (DEA) allowed only enough controlled drug to be signed out for the patient being euthanized, meaning if multiple animals required help in a single day, the veterinary team was required to return to the office to obtain more euthanasia solution each time. For better or worse, mobile veterinarians were simply unable to match the DEA's command and found themselves practicing illegally for years. In fact, when the law came up for public comment, the strongest collective voice came from veterinarians providing frequent euthanasia, the rationale being it is always best to be prepared as a matter of animal welfare.

Come what may of the inherent challenges with home euthanasia, those who offer it share how rewarding the work is. The trend will likely be toward more home services in the coming years. AAHA created the End of Life Accreditation Standards in 2020 to provide accreditation for hospital-based and mobile veterinarians who specialize in end-of-life work. The purpose of these standards is to ensure veterinary teams are practicing high-quality medicine outside of the hospital setting and to raise the bar for best practices in euthanasia and animal hospice/palliative care.

As the trend for home euthanasia grows, so does the need for neutral euthanasia settings. A client wishing to avoid the home setting, the hospital, or the local animal shelter for euthanasia is left with few alternatives. The Euthanasia Center is a budding concept that offers a safe, nonthreatening space for families to bring pets ready for the "last gift." The first one of known record is in Loveland, Colorado. Started in early 2009, it features 2 comfort rooms, a memorial garden, a quiet tone of color and sound and is fully carpeted. Today, although Euthanasia (only) Centers are still uncommon, pet crematories and veterinary hospitals are seeing the value of these neutral spaces. In recent years, I have toured numerous pet crematories with designed comfort rooms for viewings and euthanasia services. In Grand Junction, Colorado, there is a veterinary hospital that converted a next door building into a Euthanasia Center. If a patient needs the procedure, the veterinarian, patient, and grieving family travel next door for increased peace and quiet, and no memories of death will linger in the main hospital for any family member returning with the next pet. In Cincinnati, Ohio, the specialty end-of-life service Angel's Paws combines multiple offerings together. Opened in 2009, Angel's Paws provides hospice care, euthanasia, cremation, pet loss support, and retail space all under 1 roof. In each of these settings, the goal is the same: making the final moments as serene and stress free as possible. They are the manifestation of compassion through architecture and décor.

HOSPICE AND EUTHANASIA

Animal hospice and palliative medicine is a developing area of veterinary medicine with impact on euthanasia, in particular, regarding when euthanasia is chosen. As options increase and clients become aware of more choices to prolong their pet's life in a comfortable manner, euthanasia is likely to be chosen later rather than sooner, if at all. Historically, a patient became sick or advanced age took over, leading a pet owner to choose euthanasia to avoid suffering. Using strong medical approaches for pain management, infection control, and other maladies that occur as death approaches, death through euthanasia can be staved off. It is common to see euthanasia avoided for months to years, whereas in the past, the pet may have been euthanized much earlier in the disease trajectory. A familiar concept in euthanasia-centric work is to assist pets by being proactive with euthanasia instead of reactive, meaning it is better to prevent suffering and not risk a crisis-like event. Hospice and palliative care help reduce the risk of suffering leading to extended life in many cases. In situations wherein a pet owner does not want to euthanize their pet, under any circumstance, palliative sedation can be used to deliver passive euthanasia.[14] Ethically, the veterinary team must decide if euthanasia is warranted and advocate on behalf of their patients by facilitating open and honest communication with pet owners.

THE FUTURE OF EUTHANASIA

We have looked over much of the past, leading us to what is in the future for companion animal euthanasia. With increasing exploration of best practices, there already exist numerous studies investigating new drugs, techniques, team management, and client support. It is likely (and I hope) we are going to see more than 1000 references by the time the next AVMA Guidelines for the Euthanasia of Animals revised document is released, including even more on companion animals. The goal is to steadily transform euthanasia to align with science and societal expectations. There is a heightened awareness right now of "good death."

Death as a Career

In 2006, I was told by a few confused friends I was crazy to build a company around only euthanasia. Back then, only a few had attempted it, and for the most part, no one even knew it was a possibility. Turns out providing a euthanasia-only service, or one with hospice and aftercare included, has proven very rewarding for thousands. Those called to this line of work often describe it as beautiful, fulfilling, and game changing. Numerous veterinarians have told me how euthanasia work saved their veterinary careers. Physical conditions, like hand tremors, that made traditional daily medical tasks impossible could be managed easier in euthanasia work. Professionals are able to build their companies around their schedule and lifestyle, while making a huge impact in their communities. It is common for home euthanasia providers to be semiretired or seeking a change of pace from the typical veterinarian hospital environment. Knowing that many people over the years would have pursued a veterinary medicine degree had it not been for the fact they had to take life, it is interesting that some might actually become a veterinarian to do just that.

Education

A study conducted in 2017 by the sociology professor, George Dickinson, at the College of Charleston demonstrated that 100% of veterinary schools in the United Kingdom and United States taught some manner of euthanasia education.[15] To be determined through another study expected in 2020, though, is what exactly is being taught. Anecdotally, conversations with practicing veterinarians around the United States shed light on how little about euthanasia they learned in school. The old paradigm, "If you can give an injection, you know what to do," was entrenched in the university culture for decades. CAETA, founded in 2017 as an international veterinary education academy, states as their mission: *To provide outstanding education in companion animal euthanasia to improve the overall experience for the pet, caregiver, and veterinary team*. CAETA was created to fill the gap in traditional veterinary medicine curriculum, ensuring that all professionals involved in the procedure have access to proper training.

Since 2010, the number of euthanasia-featured lecture sessions at conferences has skyrocketed. Leaders in the field have been actively promoting the topic at veterinary medicine conferences and beyond in social work, thanatology, bereavement, and funeral industry venues. One of the first symposiums on the topic of euthanasia and bereavement was held in 1984 (**Fig. 3**) in New York. It brought together experts of the industry in the hopes of elevating knowledge of both the procedure and the client bereavement support in clinical practice. In this new decade, it is becoming commonplace for just about every national veterinary conference to have some euthanasia-related content for a variety of species. In 2014 and 2018, the AVMA hosted the Humane Endings Symposium. These events brought together leaders in their respective euthanasia niches to share ideas and new concepts in animal welfare. It is one of the few events in the world dedicated solely to animal euthanasia.

Increasing Cost

With added value will come rising cost to clients. Based on the success of independent veterinary euthanasia services, there is strong evidence that people are willing to pay for it. Before this century, cost of euthanasia was based almost entirely on the cost of the necessary drugs/equipment and a bit of doctor time. As hospital overhead expenses increased, along with lengthening demand on staff, euthanasia fees slowly began to increase. As of today, across the United States, euthanasia fees range from complementary/free to $500. Charges appear dependent on such things as long-term client relationships, drug expense, time allotted for the appointment, staff assistance, memorial products, and location. It is still common for veterinary teams to waive the cost of euthanasia for patients they have known and cared for.

Mobile euthanasia tends to be more expensive, and although there is no hard data to compare exact pricing trends, the average cost of the appointments today ranges from $100 to $500 depending on the region of the country. Although the higher expense can bring financial hardship to some clients, the higher cost is necessary for the veterinary teams performing it. Travel, fuel, insurance, and a reduced daily appointment volume lead mobile services to elevate the price to maintain a viable compassionate enterprise. The same can be true of euthanasia carried out in hospitals, minus the cost of travel. Euthanasia done well, with proper

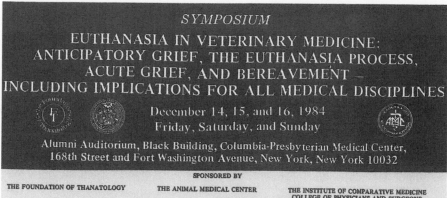

PROGRAM

FRIDAY (Evening)
6:00 P.M. to 10:00 P.M.
OVERVIEW

10 P.M. to 11:00 P.M.
SOCIAL HOUR

SATURDAY
8:00 A.M. to 12:00 P.M
EUTHANASIA IN VETERINARY MEDICINE
THE BEREAVEMENT CHRONOLOGY
OF EUTHANASIA

LUNCH – 12 :00 P.M. to 1:00 P.M.

1:00 P.M. to 3:30 P.M.
EUTHANASIA ISSUES I

3:30 P.M. to 6:00 P.M.
WORKSHOPS

6:00 P.M. to 7:00 P.M.
DINNER
(on your own)

7:00 P.M. to 10:30 P.M.
EUTHANASIA ISSUES II

SUNDAY
8:30 A.M. to 12:00 P.M.
EUTHANASIA PRACTICE PROBLEMS
AND CLIENT RELATIONS

LUNCH – 12:00 to 1:00 P.M.

1:00 P.M. to 3:00 P.M.
EUTHANASIA CASE STUDIES
(Presented to Panel)

3:00 P.M. to 5:00 P.M.
IMPLICATIONS FOR CARE
AND PROFESSIONAL PRACTICE

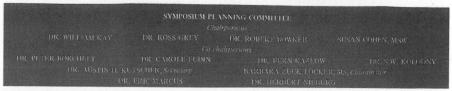

Fig. 3. Euthanasia symposium cover, 1984. (*Courtesy of* the Massachusetts MSPCA-Angell, Boston, MA; with permission.)

focus given to grief support and gentle handling of the patient, has become a specialty.

SUMMARY

As we enter into the next decade of the twenty-first century, it is clear that euthanasia is evolving. Although many veterinary teams find themselves still back in the 1970s using older outdated protocols, those paying attention to the Good Death Revolution are adapting for the betterment of pet, client, and veterinary team. Veterinary wellness has taken center stage and, with euthanasia as prevalent as ever, dedication to a gentle and meaningful experience means personnel walk away feeling valued and fulfilled. If euthanasia is deemed the most appropriate medical course, focus is then best laid on preplanning, good communication, proper technique, and compassion. When veterinary teams adhere to these, the takeaway becomes a job well done, wherein an animal is relieved of any and all suffering. It is time to free euthanasia from the stigma of failure. The gentle act can be a port in the storm.

DISCLOSURE

The author has nothing to disclose.

REFERENCES

1. Langner P. Symbolic, historical, and cultural aspects of animal euthanasia. In: Kay W, Cohen S, Fudin C, et al, editors. Euthanasia of the companion animal. Philadelphia: The Charles Press; 1988. p. 49.
2. Rollin B. Animal rights and human morality. New York: Prometheus Books; 1992. p. 222.
3. Morris P. Blue juice. Philadelphia: Temple University Press; 2012. p. 10.
4. Pierce J. The last walk. Chicago: The University of Chicago Press; 2012. p. 13.
5. Van Hooff A. Ancient euthanasia: 'good death' and the doctor in the Graeco-Roman World. Soc Sci Med 2004;58:975–85.
6. Dowbiggin I. A concise history of euthanasia; life, death, God, and medicine. Plymouth (England): Rowman and Littlefield Publishers; 2005. p. 23, 49-50.
7. AVMA 2013 Guidelines for the Euthanasia of Animals. p. 6, 10. Available at: https://www.avma.org/KB/Policies/Documents/euthanasia.pdf. Accessed September 18, 2019.
8. Definition of dysthanasia. Available at: https://en.wikipedia.org/wiki/Dysthanasia_(animal). Accessed September 10, 2019.
9. Merriam-Webster. Definition of euphemism. Available at: https://www.merriam-webster.com/dictionary/euphemism. Accessed September 1, 2019.
10. Letellier P. History and definition of a word. In: Council of Europe, editor. Euthanasia – ethical and human aspects. Germany: Council of Europe; 2003. p. 18 (1).
11. AVMA euthanasia laws by state. Available at: https://www.avma.org/Advocacy/StateAndLocal/Documents/Euthanasia_Laws.pdf. Accessed September 23, 2019.
12. Jones AW. Perspectives in drug discovery. Ln: essays on the history and development of pharmaceutical substances. Stockholm, Sweden: Dept of Forensic Genetics and Toxicology; 2010. p. 20.
13. Harris, J. From England to resurrection; acceptance and resolution of personal grief and its application to client care. In: Proceedings from euthanasia in veterinary medicine symposium. New York, December 14–16, 1984. p. 8.
14. Shearer T. Pet hospice and palliative care protocols. In: Shearer T, editor. VCNA small animal practice, palliative medicine and hospice care, vol. 41. Philadelphia: Elsevier; 2011. p. 512.
15. Dickinson GE. US and UK veterinary medicine schools: emphasis on end-of-life issues. Mortality 2019;24(1):61–71.

The Science of Transitional States of Consciousness and Euthanasia

Robert E. Meyer, DVM

KEYWORDS

- EEG - BOLD MRI - Sensory evoked potentials - Consciousness - Connectedness
- Responsiveness - Unconsciousness

KEY POINTS

- The transition from awake and conscious to an unconscious state can best be conceptualized as a nonlinear continuum.
- The interrelationships between consciousness, connectedness, and responsiveness determine individual awareness.
- Physical movements can occur in the presence of electroencephalograhic burst suppression; an electroencephalograhic pattern always associated with unconsciousness.
- Although sedatives, hypnotics, and tranquilizers administered in sufficient quantity can produce a sleep-like state, humans sedated or immobilized solely with these agents may recall connected awareness of their environment; the same is likely true for animals.
- Measures of brain electrical or metabolic activity are limited in their ability to provide defin itive answers as to exact onset of unconsciousness and do not provide information on the information transfer required for awareness of external stimuli.

INTRODUCTION

Euthanasia is defined as ending the life of an individual animal in a way that minimizes or eliminates pain and distress.[1] As veterinary professionals, our goal is to ensure the process, from awake and aware to fully unconscious and unaware, seems as if the animal simply goes to sleep. In doing so, we provide compassionate and humane care to animals in their last moments as well as peace of mind for our clients. In companion animal practice, this is usually accomplished through preprocedural sedation before the administration of a lethal overdose of an injectable anesthetic, or less frequently, an inhaled anesthetic. The accurate assessment of loss of consciousness is important in this context, for both the reporting of studies aimed at refining euthanasia methods, as well as for the practical assessment of welfare in the clinical environment.

Veterinary Anesthesiology, College of Veterinary Medicine, PO Box 6100, Campus Mailstop 9825, 240 Wise Center Drive, Mississippi State, MS 39762-6100, USA
E-mail address: robert.meyer@msstate.edu

Vet Clin Small Anim 50 (2020) 503–511
https://doi.org/10.1016/j.cvsm.2019.12.002
0195-5616/20/© 2019 Elsevier Inc. All rights reserved.

vetsmall.theclinics.com

Although the transition from conscious to unconscious may seem to be quite binary, the transition is better conceptualized as a nonlinear continuum. Loss of consciousness may occur at substantially different rates owing to several factors, such that the suitability of any particular agent or method depends on whether an animal experiences pain or distress before actual loss of consciousness. But when exactly is consciousness lost and how best to determine that point? The goal of this article is to review our understanding of loss of consciousness within the context of companion animal euthanasia.

Shortly after the breakthrough 1846 report on the use of ether anesthesia by William Morton as an adjunct to human surgery at the Harvard Medical School, Edward Mayhew published his observations in animals:

> The results of these trials are not calculated to inspire any very sanguine hopes. We cannot tell whether the cries emitted are evidence of pain or not; but they are suggestive of agony to the listener, and, without testimony to the contrary, must be regarded as evidence of suffering. The process, therefore, is not calculated to attain the object for which in veterinary practice it would be most generally employed, namely, to relieve the owner from the impression that his animal was subjected to torture. In another light, it is not likely to be of much practical utility.[2]

Unlike self-reporting humans, determining the subjective experiences of animals during transitional states of consciousness can be quite difficult. One of the defining characteristics in humans undergoing anesthesia is the feeling as if one is having an out of body experience, suggesting a disconnection between one's sense of self and one's awareness of time and space.[3] We now recognize what Dr Mayhew described in his 1847 observations are the physical signs accompanying loss of consciousness that accompany the transition between an awake conscious state (anesthesia stage 1) and the state of involuntary excitement (anesthesia stage 2). However, it would be nearly 70 years before Dr Arthur Guedel formally described the 4 stages of anesthesia based on his experience administering ether anesthesia during World War I.[4] Although we cannot know for certain the subjective experiences of animals, one can speculate that disorientation during the transition from consciousness to unconsciousness may contribute to apparent signs of animal distress observed during the initial onset of anesthesia.

CONSCIOUSNESS AND UNCONSCIOUSNESS

Although one must be conscious to subjectively experience pain and distress,[5] defining the exact moment when unconsciousness occurs in animals is quite difficult. In humans, the onset of anesthetic-induced unconsciousness continues to be functionally defined by loss of appropriate response to spoken verbal command.[6] Similarly, in animals loss of consciousness has been functionally defined by loss of the righting reflex (LORR), also called loss of position (LOP).[7,8] This definition, introduced with the introduction of general anesthesia in 1846, is still quite useful because it is an easily observable, integrated, whole animal response applicable to a wide variety of species.

The interrelationships between consciousness, connectedness, and responsiveness determine individual awareness during transitional states[9,10]: *Consciousness* is a subjective experience characterized by connectedness and awareness of the environment and to external stimuli. During wakefulness, we are conscious, connected to the environment, and responsive. Consciousness depends on the integrity of the corticothalamic networks. *Connectedness* is defined as an awareness of the external environment and to external stimuli and depends on unperturbed norepinephrinergic signaling and continued integration of information in corticothalamic circuits. *Responsiveness* is defined as spontaneous or goal-directed movements and depends on subcortical and spinal cord networks. *Unconsciousness*, defined as a loss of individual awareness to the environment and to external stimuli, occurs when information received by the cerebral cortex is reduced or the ability to integrate information is inhibited or blocked. Unconsciousness represents the graded, nonlinear collapse of multiple interconnected neural states.[11,12]

Consciousness is common during both sleep and anesthesia.[9] Consciousness can be disconnected (when not aware of the environment; eg, dreaming during sleep or during general anesthesia) or connected (eg, wakeful, where experiences can be triggered by environmental stimuli).[10]

During general anesthesia, consciousness is not necessarily associated with connectedness, responsiveness, or even recall.[9] According to information integration theory, consciousness requires the integration of scattered information processed in different brain areas.[13,14] Anesthetics produce an unconsciousness state by preventing connectedness (blocking interactions among specialized brain regions) or by decreasing available information (shrinking the number of activity patterns available to cortical networks) received by the cerebral cortex or equivalent structure or structures. Besides inducing behavioral unresponsiveness, a key goal of general anesthesia is to prevent the experience of surgery (connected consciousness) by inducing either unconsciousness or a state of disconnected consciousness from the environment.[10]

PHYSICAL MOVEMENT IN THE CONTEXT OF UNCONSCIOUSNESS

Vocalization or physical movements are often interpreted as unequivocal evidence of consciousness. Physical responses observed during the induction and maintenance of anesthesia, including reflexive movements, eye globe rotation, general muscle tone, and autonomic activity, have been traditionally taught and used in both humans and veterinary patients as signs of consciousness and used to monitor depth of anesthesia. These physical responses are now considered to be unreliable when assessing depth of anesthesia because their interpretation is based on subjective evaluation of autonomic reflexes and muscle activity. Once consciousness is lost at the onset of LORR/LOP, subsequently observed behaviors such as seizures, vocalization, reflex struggling, breath holding, and tachypnea are interpreted as signs of the excitement phase of anesthesia or stage 2, which by definition lasts from loss of consciousness to the onset of a regular breathing pattern.[15] Although unpleasant and distressing to the observer, these are not welfare issues because they occur after consciousness is lost. Further, observable physical responses such as eye globe rotation, reflexes, and muscle tone are affected in substantially different ways by different anesthetics.[16]

Similarly, patient movement occurring during anesthesia and surgical procedures has traditionally been interpreted as indicating an animal is underanesthetized. Human and animal studies confirm the onset of amnesia and blockade of conscious awareness at less than one-half the anesthetic concentration required to abolish physical movement.[8] It is now accepted that nonpurposeful movement in response to noxious stimulation in unconscious anesthetized animals is due to spinally mediated reflex activity and is abolished primarily by means of anesthetic action within the spinal cord rather than the cerebral cortex.[8] Physical movements can even occur in the presence of electroencephalograhic burst suppression, a drug-induced or brain damaged electroencephalogram (EEG) pattern always associated with unconsciousness. Indeed, spontaneous and often complex movement can occur in unconscious, decerebrate, or spinally transected humans and animals owing to neural circuits at the level of the brainstem and spinal cord not requiring connection with the cerebral cortex.[8] Thus, vocalization and nonpurposeful movements observed after LORR/LOP, although unwelcome in the euthanasia context, are not necessarily signs of conscious perception by an animal.

Conversely, immobility or unresponsiveness to noxious stimulation does not necessarily imply unconsciousness or lack of awareness.[10] A common characteristic of both sedatives and tranquillizers (eg, D2 dopamine antagonists, namely, phenothiazines, butyrophenones; serotonin reuptake inhibitors, namely, trazodone; alpha-2 agonists, namely, xylazine, dexmedetomidine) is that arousal to a conscious state can occur with sufficient stimulation, such that animals sedated or immobilized with these agents may still be arousable and aware of their environment. Although sedatives, hypnotics, and tranquilizers administered in sufficient quantity can produce a sleep-like state, humans may recall connected awareness of their environment; indeed, high doses of alpha-2 agonists (eg, dexmedetomidine) are unreliable in producing a general anesthetic state of unconsciousness in humans[17] or animals.[18] Although combinations such as dexmedetomidine and butorphanol with or without acepromazine are commonly used in veterinary medicine for procedures such as laceration repair, nerve blocks or tissue infiltration with local anesthetics are still necessary to prevent nociception and responsiveness. In addition to sedative and tranquilizer combinations, agents capable of producing a state of general anesthesia, such as gamma amino butyric acid type A agonists (eg, pentobarbital, alfaxalone, propofol) or N-methyl-D-aspartate antagonists (eg, ketamine, tiletamine) should be considered as necessary components of the euthanasia process to unambiguously ensure that animals are truly unconscious or disconnected from their environment.

ELECTROPHYSIOLOGIC AND METABOLIC MEASURES OF UNCONSCIOUSNESS

Measurements of brain electrical function have been applied to both humans and animals to more precisely define the transition to an unconscious state.[9,16,19–21] Measurements of brain electrical function include: the raw unprocessed electroencephalogram (EEG), various Fourier or power analyses of the processed EEG frequency domain (eg, total power, median frequency, and spectral edge), proprietary algorithm-based analyses such as bispectral analysis (BIS index) and Index of Consciousness, visual and auditory evoked potentials, electrocortigraphy, and low-resolution electromagnetic tomography. Although the issue in humans is preventing intraoperative awareness, in animals the issue is procedural humaneness relative to onset of unconsciousness. This task is even more difficult in animals because we cannot question them directly and must infer by observing their actions and responses.

Although measures of brain electrical or metabolic activity are often applied to determine the state of consciousness, these methods are currently acknowledged to be limited in their ability to provide definitive answers as to exact onset of either human or animal unconsciousness.[16] An EEG is not a direct measure of consciousness; it measures brain electrical activity and, although that activity changes with levels of consciousness, an EEG cannot provide definitive answers as to precise onset of human unconsciousness using the current state of the art.[6,22,23] Although consciousness must vanish at some level between behavioral unresponsiveness and the induction of a flatline EEG (indicating the cessation of the brain's electrical activity and an unconscious state), current EEG-based brain function monitors are acknowledged to be limited in their ability to definitively confirm unconsciousness, especially around the transition point.[11,20] Further, the EEG does not provide information on the presence or absence of information transfer within the brain, which is required for awareness to stimuli.[24]

The exact moment when animal unconsciousness occurs is difficult to determine based on the EEG as the changes are often gradual and unlike verbally responsive humans, there is no bright line response to spoken verbal command to delineate when consciousness is lost.[6] There are 4 different types of wave patterns in the EEG that can be distinguished based on their respective frequencies and that are related to the state of consciousness: δ (0–4 Hz), θ (4–8 Hz), α (8–12 Hz), and β (>12 Hz) waves. Both δ and θ (slow wave) activity is related to sleep or reduced consciousness. Alpha wave activity is prominent in subjects that are conscious, but mentally inactive (closing eyes and relaxation) and β waves are associated with active movements and increased alertness.[21]

Consciousness is characterized by high-frequency (α and β), low-amplitude waves, and an increase in low-frequency activity is accompanied by an increase in amplitude as animals lose consciousness.[25] However, although the onset of slow-frequency high-amplitude waves is used to infer loss of consciousness, these waves may also be observed during wakefulness in both rodents[26] and humans.[27] In isoflurane-anesthetized rats, where decreased frequency and increased δ power was observed at the loss of righting reflex, an EEG similar to the awake state was produced when the rat was rolled on its side, regardless of whether the rat could right itself.[28] In the same study, paw pinch and tail clamp produced similar signs of EEG activation even during deep anesthesia when EEG burst suppression dominated the EEG. The interpretation of these observations as to the conscious or unconscious state was profoundly influenced by the method of EEG analysis (chaos analysis vs traditional Fourier transformation analysis). Further, it is difficult to compare EEG values between studies and species owing to variations in experimental conditions and equipment, anesthesia, electrode placements, skull thickness, overlying muscles, interindividual variability, number of EEG stages used in the assessment of unconsciousness, and acquisition artifacts.[21]

Although EEG waveform changes are correlated weakly with anesthetic depth, the EEG alone is not usually considered a sensitive or specific index of anesthetic depth. This is due to several factors, including the limited number of recognized EEG patterns and the large number of variables affecting EEG patterns. Increasing anesthetic concentration can produce different, overlapping EEG patterns depending on species and anesthetic, with progression of EEG changes depending on the relative effects of the agent on the hypnotic state.[19] EEG power spectrum varies with anesthetic choice[9,29] and existing EEG-based anesthetic depth monitors, such as bispectral analysis, are noted to be unreliable indicators of awareness in humans receiving neuromuscular blocking agents[30] as well as during N-methyl-D-aspartate receptor-based anesthesia (eg, N_2O, ketamine).[31] In humans, substantial differences in EEG reactivity are reported at the same clinical endpoint (response to spoken verbal command) with propofol, dexmedetomidine, and sevoflurane[17]; this finding has profound implications for the use of EEG in evaluation of animal consciousness in that EEG observations may not be directly comparable between different anesthetics or physical methods. EEG-based indices are currently not part of standard human anesthetic practice, largely because their use does not ensure that awareness is prevented under general anesthesia.[22,23]

Evoked potentials, such as auditory, visual, or somatosensory, measure the electrophysiologic responses of the nervous system to a variety of stimuli, where complete absence of sensory evoked potentials is definitive for lack of awareness to external stimuli. The visual evoked potential tests the function of the visual pathway from the retina to the occipital cortex. It measures the conduction of the visual pathways from the optic nerve, optic chiasm, and optic radiations to the occipital cortex. The auditory evoked potential measures the functioning of the auditory nerve and auditory pathways in the brainstem. In humans, evoked potentials are correlated with awareness to a stimulus or response to verbal commands[17,32]; however, these kinds of studies are difficult to perform in nonverbal animals. Anesthetic agents reduce evoked potentials in a continuous, rather than a binary, manner, and there is no currently accepted definition as to where sensory awareness is lost within that continuum. Evoked potentials may be present in surgically anesthetized, unconscious animals.[33] In rats, visual cortex neurons remain responsive to flash stimulation during desflurane anesthesia and reduced gamma oscillations do not correlate with unconsciousness.[34,35] Large interindividual variations in auditory evoked potential and bispectral analysis make it impossible to discriminate subtle changes of clinical state of consciousness in real time during propofol anesthesia.[36] Evoked potentials also do not provide information as to perception of internal sensations of allodynia or pain.

Blood oxygen level-dependent MRI is a multifactorial surrogate for cerebral blood flow or cerebral blood volume, both of which are actual measures of neural activity. Blood oxygen level-dependent MRI imaging exploits the presence of deoxyhemoglobin in tissues as a contrast media and provides in vivo maps of changes in brain activity triggered by pharmacologic or physiologic events. Although a blood oxygen level-dependent MRI response is generally a good surrogate measure of neuronal activity, it is based on hemodynamic changes that may not reflect actual neural activity patterns, especially during anesthesia or under pharmacologic challenge; rather, observed effects may be directly due to drug effects or indirectly through changes in autonomic activity, blood pressure, cardiac output, or respiration.[37,38] In contrast, imaging of cerebral blood flow using PET scans has been used in human volunteers during manipulation of consciousness with anesthetics combined with response to spoken verbal command[12]; the application of similar methods in animals to explore the transition between the conscious and unconsciousness state will be difficult.

So how can we assure our clients, and ourselves, that animals are not aware or suffering during euthanasia? Drawing inferences from the human experience is attractive but flawed in that subjective human experiences may not coincide with the subjective experiences of animals. We can identify whether a brain is active or inactive; however, determining the exact moment that consciousness is lost during dynamic transitional states remains difficult. We can only infer an unconscious, unresponsive state exists in animals because observed EEG patterns are similar to those observed in human studies. Although slower EEG waveform oscillations are assumed to indicate a more profound state of general anesthesia, and increasing doses of several intravenous and inhaled anesthetics eventually induce slowing in EEG oscillations, the same waveform or index value is assumed to reflect the same level of unconsciousness for all anesthetics, which is simplistic and not supported by current research. Electrical and metabolic indices of brain activity do not ensure that awareness is lost and cannot give an accurate picture of the brain's responses to anesthetics because they do not relate directly to the neurophysiology of how specific anesthetics exert their effects in the brain.

Despite decades of intensive study, using currently available methods we can only approximate the subjective experiences of animals during transitional states of consciousness. Until we have better assessment tools, behavior-based observations, such as LORR/LOP remain among our most useful guides to the onset of unconsciousness in animals. To minimize potential animal suffering and to ensure a truly unconscious or disconnected state is unambiguously achieved, a state of general anesthesia relying on gamma amino butyric acid type A agonists (eg, pentobarbital, propofol, alfaxalone) or N-methyl-ᴅ-aspartate antagonists (eg, ketamine, tiletamine) continues to be a necessary component of the companion animal euthanasia process.

DISCLOSURE

The author has no competing commercial or financial conflicts of interest to declare.

REFERENCES

1. Leary SL. American Veterinary Medical Association. AVMA guidelines for the euthanasia of animals: 2013 Edition. 2013. Available at: https://www.avma.org/KB/Policies/Documents/euthanasia.pdf. Accessed January 23, 2018.
2. Carter HE, Mayhew E. On the effects of inhalation of the fumes of æther on dogs and cats, and, by inference, on the horse; with the probable utility of such in veterinary medicine. J Small Anim Pract 1984;25(1):31–5.
3. Banks WP. Encyclopedia of consciousness, vol. 1. Cambridge (MA): Academic Press; 2009.
4. Drew BA. Arthur Guedel and the ascendance of anesthesia: a teacher, tinkerer, and transformer. J Anesth Hist 2018. https://doi.org/10.1016/j.janh.2018.08.002.
5. IASP Terminology - IASP. Available at: https://www.iasp-pain.org/terminology?navItemNumber=576#Pain. Accessed March 8, 2019.
6. Juel BE, Romundstad L, Kolstad F, et al. Distinguishing anesthetized from awake state in patients: a new approach using one second segments of raw EEG. Front Hum Neurosci 2018;12. https://doi.org/10.3389/fnhum.2018.00040.
7. Hondrickx JFA, Eger EI, Sonner JM, et al. Is synergy the rule? a review of anesthetic interactions producing hypnosis and immobility. Anesth Analg 2008; 107(2):494.
8. Antognini JF, Barter L, Carstens E. Movement as an index of anesthetic depth in humans and experimental animals. 2005. Available at: http://www.ingentaconnect.com/content/aalas/cm/2005/00000055/00000005/art00001; jsessionid=cfba6s1sbi8o3.x-ic-live-02. Accessed June 5, 2018.
9. Marchant N, Sanders R, Sleigh J, et al. How electroencephalography serves the anesthesiologist. Clin EEG Neurosci 2014;45(1):22–32.
10. Sanders RD, Tononi G, Laureys S, et al. Unresponsiveness ≠ unconsciousness. Anesthesiology 2012;116(4):946–59.
11. Alkire MT, Hudetz AG, Tononi G. Consciousness and anesthesia. Science 2008; 322(5903):876–80.
12. Långsjö JW, Alkire MT, Kaskinoro K, et al. Returning from oblivion: imaging the neural core of consciousness. J Neurosci 2012;32(14):4935–43.
13. Soddu A, Vanhaudenhuyse A, Bahri MA, et al. Identifying the default-mode component in spatial IC analyses of patients with disorders of consciousness. Hum Brain Mapp 2012;33(4):778–96.
14. Cauda F, Micon BM, Sacco K, et al. Disrupted intrinsic functional connectivity in the vegetative state. J Neurol Neurosurg Psychiatry 2009;80(4):429–31.
15. Muir WW. Considerations for general anesthesia. Lumb Jones' Vet Anesth Analg. 4th edition. Ames (IA): Blackwell; 2007. p. 7–30.
16. Silva A, Antunes L. Electroencephalogram-based anaesthetic depth monitoring in laboratory animals. Lab Anim 2012;46(2):85–94.

17. Kaskinoro K, Maksimow A, Georgiadis S, et al. Electroencephalogram reactivity to verbal command after dexmedetomidine, propofol and sevoflurane-induced unresponsiveness. Anaesthesia 2015;70(2):190–204.

18. Dewell R, Bergamasco L, Kelly C, et al. Clinical study to assess the level of consciousness/general anesthesia following the administration of high doses of xylazine hydrochloride in cattle. Anim Ind Rep 2014;660(1). Available at: https://lib.dr.iastate.edu/ans_air/vol660/iss1/13. Accessed January 13, 2020.

19. March PA, Muir WW. Bispectral analysis of the electroencephalogram: a review of its development and use in anesthesia. Vet Anaesth Analg 2005;32(5): 241–55.

20. Mashour GA, Avidan MS. Intraoperative awareness: controversies and non-controversies. Br J Anaesth 2015;115(Supplement 1):i20–6.

21. Verhoeven MTW, Gerritzen MA, Hellebrekers LJ, et al. Indicators used in livestock to assess unconsciousness after stunning: a review. Animal 2015;9(2):320–30.

22. Purdon PL, Sampson A, Pavone KJ, et al. Clinical electroencephalography for anesthesiologists: part I: background and basic signatures. Anesthesiology 2015; 123(4):937–60.

23. Crosby G, Culley DJ. Processed electroencephalogram and depth of anesthesia window to nowhere or into the brain? Anesthesiology 2012;116(2):235–7.

24. Sherman SM. Thalamus plays a central role in ongoing cortical functioning. Nat Neurosci 2016;19(4):533–41.

25. Seth AK, Baars BJ, Edelman DB. Criteria for consciousness in humans and other mammals. Conscious Cogn 2005;14(1):119–39.

26. Vyazovskiy VV, Olcese U, Hanlon EC, et al. Local sleep in awake rats. Nature 2011;472(7344):443–7.

27. Huber R, Ghilardi MF, Massimini M, et al. Local sleep and learning. Nature 2004; 430(6995):78–81.

28. Maciver B, Bland BH. Chaos analysis of EEG during isoflurane-induced loss of righting in rats. Front Syst Neurosci 2014;8. https://doi.org/10.3389/fnsys.2014.00203.

29. Solovey G, Alonso LM, Yanagawa T, et al. Loss of consciousness is associated with stabilization of cortical activity. J Neurosci 2015;35(30):10866–77.

30. Schuller PJ, Newell S, Strickland PA, et al. Response of bispectral index to neuromuscular block in awake volunteers. Br J Anaesth 2015;115(suppl_1):i95–103.

31. Kuhlmann L, Liley DTJ. Assessing nitrous oxide effect using electroencephalographically-based depth of anesthesia measures cortical state and cortical input. J Clin Monit Comput 2018;32(1):173–88.

32. Palva S, Linkenkaer-Hansen K, Näätänen R, et al. Early neural correlates of conscious somatosensory perception. J Neurosci 2005;25(21):5248–58.

33. Musall S, Haiss F, Weber B, et al. Deviant processing in the primary somatosensory cortex. Cereb Cortex 2017;27(1):863–76.

34. Hudetz AG, Vizuete JA, Imas OA. Desflurane selectively suppresses long-latency cortical neuronal response to flash in the rat. Anesthesiology 2009; 111(2):231–9.

35. Imas OA, Ropella KM, Ward BD, et al. Volatile anesthetics enhance flash-induced γ oscillations in rat visual cortex. Anesthesiology 2005;102(5):937–47.

36. Barr G, Anderson RE, Jakobsson JG. A study of bispectral analysis and auditory evoked potential indices during propofol-induced hypnosis in volunteers: the effect of an episode of wakefulness on explicit and implicit memory. Anaesthesia 2001;56(9):888–92.

37. Baudelet C, Gallez B. Effect of anesthesia on the signal intensity in tumors using BOLD-MRI: comparison with flow measurements by Laser Doppler flowmetry and oxygen measurements by luminescence-based probes. Magn Reson Imaging 2004;22(7):905–12.
38. Steward CA, Marsden CA, Prior MJW, et al. Methodological considerations in rat brain BOLD contrast pharmacological MRI. Psychopharmacology (Berl) 2005; 180(4):687–704.

The Pathophysiology of Dying

Beth Marchitelli, DVM, MS

KEYWORDS

- Pathophysiology of death/dying veterinary medicine
- Mechanisms of death veterinary medicine • Bichat's triad • Somatic death
- Cellular death

KEY POINTS

- The pathophysiology of dying for veterinary patients has historically warranted less attention than normal and abnormal physiologic mechanisms geared to the preservation of life.
- Bichat's triad, with the addition of metabolic and toxic causes of death, provides a framework for understanding the pathophysiology of death in veterinary patients.
- Acute death initiated by specific causes in human patients can serve as models for understanding death in veterinary patients under certain conditions.
- The prevalence of euthanasia for veterinary patients obscures pathophysiologic processes that occur as pets reach the final stages of death.
- The complex interplay of environmental factors and individual differences shape the pathophysiology of death for each veterinary patient.

INTRODUCTION

In veterinary medicine, the pathophysiology of dying has received less attention than normal and abnormal physiologic processes, because these processes relate directly to keeping pets alive. Additionally, because many veterinary patients are euthanized, the pathophysiologic process of dying, as it occurs outside of the context of euthanasia, has warranted less extensive scrutiny both academically and clinically. In contrast, in the United States the vast majority of the human population dies without formal medical aid in dying. Many human patients do benefit from hospice and palliative care services as they near death. Thus, human medicine has a more sophisticated and nuanced understanding of the pathophysiology of dying as a result of direct experience and experimental evidence imparted (coincidentally) from animal models. Studies are numerous, with contributions from the fields of resuscitation science, organ transplant medicine, forensic science, mortuary science,

4 Paws Farewell: Mobile Pet Hospice, Palliative Care and Home Euthanasia, Asheville, NC, USA
E-mail address: bmarchitelli@hotmail.com

Vet Clin Small Anim 50 (2020) 513–524
https://doi.org/10.1016/j.cvsm.2019.12.003
0195-5616/20/© 2019 Elsevier Inc. All rights reserved.

emergency medicine, and hospice and palliative medicine. The pathophysiology of dying is determined by the inciting cause or causes, which are in turn influenced by such factors as individual variation, rate of disease progression, and access to medical resources. Because of this complexity, developing a general model of dying in veterinary medicine proves difficult. Extrapolating from the human literature in cases where dying has occurred acutely and has been propagated by specific mechanisms (cardiac, respiratory, central nervous system, and metabolic) provides insight and understanding that may be more directly applicable to veterinary patients. This article proposes mechanisms of dying for veterinary patients that succumb to death by way of primary insult to the cardiac, respiratory, and central nervous systems. Death caused by metabolic derangement; dehydration or a combination of the two, are also discussed. Last, and most pertinent for many veterinary patients, the pathophysiology of dying, in the context of euthanasia induced by sodium pentobarbital is analyzed.

BICHAT'S TRIAD IN VETERINARY MEDICINE

In forensic science, the mechanisms of death have historically been understood by way of Bichat's triad. Bichat's triad consists of 3 general modes of death: syncope (cardiac impairment), coma (insult to the cerebrum, brainstem, or nervous system), and asphyxia (respiratory impairment).[1] Mechanisms of death can also be understood more generally, culminating as a result of impaired oxygen delivery to the tissues, resulting in hypoxia and subsequent cell death. For this paradigm, one has to assume that impaired oxygen delivery to the tissues results in cardiac arrest; however, the exact pathway to this end is less clear.

For the purposes of applicability to veterinary medicine, the framework of Bichat's triad has been used with the addition of a fourth category: metabolic or toxic insult (Fig. 1). The proposed mechanisms and specific diseases chosen for this article are by no means exhaustive. In addition, insult to 1 body system often leads to failure in another; thus, the physiologic processes discussed are interrelated and have much overlap in contributing to cardiac arrest. Division of specific disease processes into the categories described elsewhere in this article only serves as a framework for understanding. Future scientific investigation and study, pertaining to end-stage disease processes in veterinary medicine, is warranted to advance our knowledge in this area and thus guide recommendations for adequate supportive care aimed at sufficiently alleviating suffering.

MECHANISMS OF DEATH: THE BRAIN AND THE CENTRAL NERVOUS SYSTEM
Brain Tumors: Meningiomas

Exploring injury to vital structures in the brain and central nervous system is a good starting point, because insults to other body systems (cardiovascular, respiratory, metabolic) can secondarily alter blood flow or oxygen delivery to the brain resulting in similar mechanisms of impairment and subsequent death.

Meningiomas are the most common primary brain tumors in both dogs and cats.[2,3] In humans, meningiomas represented 30% of all intracranial neoplasms.[4] Although sudden death is rare in humans with meningiomas because most cases progress slowly with a predictable course of neurologic clinical signs, it has been described.[4] In an article by Gitto and colleagues[4] in 2018, sudden death related to meningiomas in humans was hypothesized to be related to increased intracranial pressure (ICP), acute hemorrhage, compression of vital nerve centers or direct invasion of vital nerve tissue (Fig. 2).

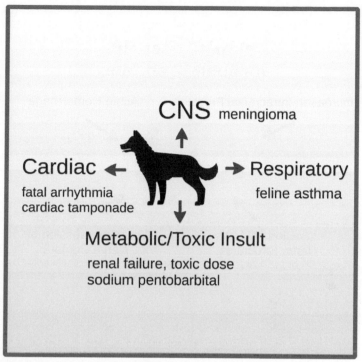

Fig. 1. Bichat's triad in veterinary medicine.

Increased Intracranial pressure

Increased ICP can be caused by cerebral edema, which is a common finding in intracranial meningiomas in humans.[5] Peritumoral edema can comprise an area several times larger than the tumor itself.[4] The physical presence of the tumor can impair or impede blood flow mechanically, resulting in focal hypoxia, cerebral edema, and increased ICP. Depending on the location of the tumor, direct obstruction of the cerebral spinal fluid can also cause elevated ICP.[4,6] When compensation for increased ICP is exhausted, cerebral herniation can occur. This process can contribute to compression and impairment of vital centers in the brain stem controlling respiratory drive, namely, the reticular formation, resulting in respiratory arrest and subsequent cardiac arrest.[6–8] Increased ICP may occur independently or in conjunction with the mechanisms described elsewhere in this article.

Direct Compression of Vital Nerve Centers

For meningiomas that are located adjacent to the brain stem, direct compression of the reticular formation by the tumor can lead to cardiac arrhythmias, respiratory dysfunction, and subsequent death. Tumors compressing the hypothalamus can impair autonomic control. Structures of the hypothalamus play a key role in cardiac regulation and, thus, if disabled can lead to sudden cardiac arrest.[9] Most meningiomas in cats are located rostral to the tentorium of the cerebellum, making indirect compression more likely in these species.[10] Death that results from direct compression of vital structures is determined by the location of the tumor and its ability to create forces sufficient to impede nerve conduction and regulation.

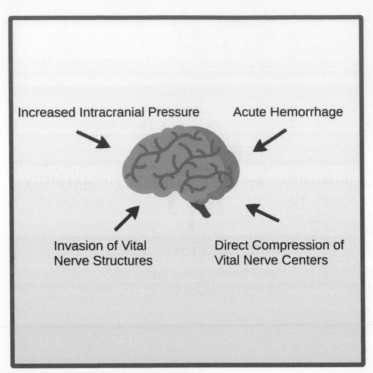

Fig. 2. Mechanisms of acute death: brain tumors.

Acute Hemorrhage

Spontaneous intratumoral hemorrhage arising from meningiomas in humans is rare; however, it has been reported to occur in 1.3% to 2.4% of cases, with death occurring in 28% to 50% of cases.[11] In 2010, Martin-Vaquero and colleagues[12] described a case of acute intratumoral hemorrhage in a dog. The etiology of acute hemorrhage in these cases is unknown; however, several mechanisms have been proposed. For instance, cerebral edema and acute hemorrhage can cause increased ICP, resulting in impairment of vital centers in the brain stem leading to death. The incidence of intratumoral hemorrhage in dogs and cats with meningiomas is unknown at this time; however, hemorrhage could play a role in sudden death in these species.

Direct Invasion of Vital Centers by Tumor Cells

Meningiomas do not generally infiltrate surrounding brain tissue, but malignant forms can do so. Consistent with the described mechanisms, invasion of vital structures within the brain stem by tumor cells can result in death. Secondary compression perpetuated by infiltration of brain tissue elsewhere resulting in cerebral edema and elevated ICP can compress vital centers in the brain stem, leading to respiratory depression and cardiac arrest. In addition, invasion of adjacent blood vessels by malignant tumor cells can result in acute hemorrhage, leading to elevated ICP and sudden death.[13]

Increased ICP, acute hemorrhage, and compression or invasion of vital nerve centers may occur independently or simultaneously in contributing to acute death in dogs and cats with meningiomas. The following is an example of these mechanisms at play in a cat. This example illustrates how clinical signs seen in patients can be explained by underlying pathophysiologic mechanisms.

Case Example: Meningioma

Max: signalment: 13-year-old male neutered domestic short hair cat

Max presented to his regular veterinarian with progressive signs of altered mentation and partial seizure activity.[14] A computed tomography scan revealed an intracranial tumor located along the meninges of the third ventricle of the diencephalon, suspected to be a meningioma. Palliative care was elected and surgery was declined. Over the next several months, Max exhibited progressive signs of abnormal mentation, partial seizure activity, poor appetite, and weight loss. Three months after Max first presented to his regular veterinarian, he experienced an acute episode of stupor, followed by Cheyne Stokes respiration, which progressed to apnea and then cardiac arrest.

In this case, Max lost consciousness owing to increased ICP affecting the brain stem. This compression progressed, descending along structures in the medulla leading to Cheyne Stokes respiration, apnea, and resultant cardiac arrest. This case illustrates 1 example of the possible mechanisms contributing to acute death in cats with meningiomas.

Mechanisms of Death: Cardiac Impairment

Fatal arrhythmias

Boxers are predisposed to arrhythmogenic right ventricular cardiomyopathy, which is akin to arrhythmogenic cardiomyopathy in humans.[15] Both diseases can result in sudden death. In a study by Basso and colleagues[16] (2004), of 9 Boxers that died suddenly, 6 experienced cardiac arrhythmias.

Pulseless electrical activity, ventricular fibrillation, and other serious arrhythmias can proceed to cardiac arrest. After a prolonged period of inefficient circulatory capacity and subsequent inadequate oxygen delivery, cardiac myocytes enter into a period of metabolic derangement.[17] This cascade renders the heart, as a whole, to quiescence. Literature in resuscitation science is robust, describing specific biochemical mechanisms and phases of cardiac arrest in the hopes of applying interventions to reverse this process in humans.[18–20] Fatal arrhythmias in humans are thought to lead to cardiac arrest as a result of dysfunctional cardiac myocytes affected by tissue ischemia and hypoxia.

Cardiac tamponade

A similar pathway can occur in cases of cardiac tamponade, eventually leading to cardiac myocyte ischemia, hypoxia, and exhaustion. Unlike fatal arrhythmias, which cause cardiac arrest owing to aberrant electrical function, cardiac tamponade impairs oxygen delivery mechanically. Interestingly, in human medicine, the extent of pericardial effusion determines the presence of pulsus paradoxus. Pulsus paradoxus is defined as a change in arterial blood pressure during inspiration that is greater than 10 mm Hg.[21] In veterinary patients, this change manifests as a weak or absent palpable pulse during inspiration. In human patients, if cardiac output is severely compromised (such as in cardiac tamponade), pulsus paradoxus is likely.[22]

The majority of cardiac tumors in dogs have been identified as hemangiosarcoma (69%).[23] A range of between 8.7% to 25% of cases of splenic hemangiosarcoma have been reported to have a right atrial mass.[24] Dogs diagnosed with splenic hemangiosarcoma could deteriorate from hemorrhage originating from the spleen, an associated right atrial mass, or from diffuse metastatic disease. In cases of hemorrhage associated with a right atrial mass, pericardial effusion and cardiac tamponade can contribute to death.

Case Example: Atrial and Splenic Hemangiosarcoma

Charlie: signalment: 9-year-old male neutered Great Pyrenees

Charlie was diagnosed with presumptive hemangiosarcoma of the spleen and right atria. He declined acutely while at home, with clinical signs of dyspnea, weakness, and collapse. Over several hours, his breathing became labored, he lost consciousness (when central systolic blood pressure drops below 60 mm Hg, unconsciousness ensues),[25] and pulsus paradoxus was noted. Charlie died shortly thereafter. Before his death, he experienced several agonal breaths.

In this case, Charlie likely experienced cardiac tamponade, caused by pericardial effusion. The heart muscle eventually failed owing to decreased cardiac output, causing cardiac myocyte ischemia and hypoxia. Agonal respiration is hypothesized to be a response to severe hypoxemia, initiated experimentally when arterial oxygen tension is less than 5 mm Hg.[26]

Congestive Heart Failure

Death from congestive heart failure in veterinary patients is multifactorial. Most simplistically, a cardiac component and respiratory component contribute to patient demise; thus, it is difficult to classify here. Hypertrophic cardiomyopathy in cats is known to cause sudden death; however, based on a study by Wilkie and colleagues[27] in 2015, the etiology is unclear. Last, dilated cardiomyopathy is also known to cause sudden death; however, like the aforementioned cardiac diseases, the etiology is likely related to multiple factors. A discussion of all causes of cardiac death and their mechanisms is beyond the scope of this article. The cases chosen were simplified to illustrate possible pathophysiologic mechanisms. The diseases selected were based on the availability of research and data supportive of such processes in human medicine.

MECHANISMS OF DEATH: RESPIRATORY IMPAIRMENT
Feline Asthma

The etiology of sudden death in humans from fatal episodes of asthma is thought to be caused by respiratory arrest leading to cardiac arrest, rather than cardiac cessation induced by cardiac arrhythmia.[28] Patients who experience a fatal episode of asthma have also been reported to have concurrent hypercapnia-induced ventilatory failure, respiratory acidosis, and overlying metabolic acidosis.[28] In human patients, warning signs predictive of decompensation include worsening dyspnea, night time waking, and wheezing.[28]

Asthma in cats is pathophysiologically similar to that in humans, with a reported incidence of 1% to 5% of all cats.[29] Unlike humans, cats exhibit cough as a common clinical sign, as opposed to humans whose chief complaint is dyspnea.[30] Feline asthma is hypothesized to be a type I hypersensitivity reaction, causing lower airway inflammation and resultant airway hyperactivity, increased mucous production, and smooth muscle hypertrophy.[30] Fatal episodes of asthma in cats are likely similar, mechanistically, to those in humans. In response to decreasing levels of oxygen and increasing levels of carbon dioxide, abnormal respiratory patterns may be a precursor to respiratory arrest.[31] Depending on the amount of oxygen available for use at the time of respiratory arrest, cardiac arrest occurs presumably when cardiac myocytes fail as a result of hypoxia. Once the heart stops contracting, the body will use up all stores of oxygen in approximately 4 minutes, and the machinery for cellular processes will start to fail.[32] Consistent with cases of fatal arrhythmias and cardiac tamponade, cardiac arrest in cases of fatal episodes of asthma is a consequence of cardiac myocyte dysfunction and failure.

Case Example: Feline Asthma

Rosie: signalment: 8-year-old female spayed domestic short hair cat

Rosie was diagnosed with feline asthma at 2 years of age. As she aged, her symptoms increased in frequency, prompting 2 visits to the emergency clinic. One week after returning home from her last trip to the emergency clinic, Rosie experienced several bouts of coughing, open mouth breathing, and wheezing. Rosie then became laterally recumbent and unconscious. After several minutes, she exhibited 2 agonal breaths and then stopped breathing. Her heart stopped within several minutes.

In this case example, suppression of oxygen exchange at the level of the lower airways resulted in ischemia and hypoxia of the heart muscle leading to cardiac arrest. Fatal episodes of feline asthma are representative of other terminal respiratory diseases that impair oxygen delivery, eventually affecting cardiac myocytes and cardiac function. Such global hypoxia causes metabolic derangement in cellular processes in the brain and other vital organs, contributing to overall demise.

MECHANISMS OF DEATH: METABOLIC DISEASE
Renal Failure

End-stage renal failure deleteriously impacts many organ systems in the body. Specifically, uremic toxins negatively affect the central nervous system, cardiovascular system, respiratory system, and gastrointestinal system.[33] The inability to clear renal toxins also creates a proinflammatory and immunocompromised environment.[33]

In human patients, there is a strong connection between renal disease and coronary artery disease, warranting the name cardiorenal syndrome.[34] In veterinary medicine, Pouchelon and colleagues[26] coined the term cardiovascular–renal disorders in a consensus statement derived from veterinary cardiologists and nephrologists in the Journal of Small Animal Practice in 2015. Because primary renal and cardiac disease processes differ between humans and veterinary patients, a direct comparison from human medicine is challenging. There is however good evidence to establish a relationship between these 2 diseases in veterinary patients. Proposed mechanisms include renal propagated systemic hypertension leading to impaired cardiac output and arrhythmias as well as cardiac arrhythmias generated by alterations in serum potassium.[35]

In end-stage renal disease, the effects of dehydration, hypovolemia, and metabolic acidosis negatively impact multiple organ systems, including the cardiovascular, respiratory, and central nervous systems.[36] The cause of clinical signs suggestive of encephalopathy, including seizures, are unknown; however, they are hypothesized to be related to the effects of uremic toxins, impaired cerebral oxygen metabolism, elevated levels of parathyroid hormone,[37] and/or reported hypoglycemia.[38] Based on these findings, the path to ultimate demise has many interrelated constituents. Investigating contributing factors to death in cases of end-stage renal disease can instruct best supportive care measures focusing on comfort.

Case Example: Renal Failure

Rex: signalment: 17-year-old male neutered domestic short hair cat

Rex was diagnosed with chronic renal disease and hypertension at his most recent veterinary visit, prompted by his clinical decline occurring over several weeks. Rex's appetite, energy level, and water intake had been poor. Several days after his veterinary visit, his owners came home to find him on his side having a seizure. After several minutes, he extended his cervical spine and both forelimbs in a position of opisthotonus and died shortly after.

Numerous factors could have contributed to this scenario. For example, the combination of dehydration, hypovolemia, and uremic toxins could have induced a fatal arrhythmia. Rex could have also developed increased ICP resulting from impaired cerebral oxygen metabolism, leading to compression of vital structures in the brain stem.[39] This particular case incorporates many of the mechanisms discussed previously, namely, the sequelae of increased ICP and the effects of fatal arrhythmias.

MECHANISMS OF DEATH: TOXIC INSULT
Euthanasia Solution

Sodium pentobarbital is the active ingredient in available euthanasia agents in the United States. In human medicine, sodium pentobarbital can be used to induce a medical coma to help alleviate elevated ICP.[40] However, rapid intravenous administration can have several detrimental effects, including severe respiratory depression, vasodilation, and hypotension.[41]

Sodium pentobarbital is highly lipid soluble, and thus penetrates the brain readily, with cerebral blood flow as a limiting factor.[41] The exact mechanism(s) on the central nervous system is not entirely clear, but it is thought to be mediated by its effect on gamma-aminobutyric acid, the primary inhibitory neurotransmitter in the brain.[41]

In veterinary patients, when given at lethal doses intravenously, sodium pentobarbital causes rapid depression in systemic blood pressure, followed by respiratory arrest owing to suppression of the reticular formation in the medulla. This suppression of vital centers in the brain stem (reticular formation) may be related to a rapid decrease in cerebral profusion and/or direct suppression by the drug itself. As cerebral profusion pressure drops unconsciousness ensues,[42] followed by an isoelectric electric encephalogram, demonstrating the absence of electrical activity in the brain.[40,43] Several minutes after apnea, cardiac arrest ensues.[40,43] The mechanism for cardiac arrest, similar to that of acute respiratory arrest described previously, is likely ischemia, hypoxia, and the consequential inability of the heart to generate a cardiac rhythm. Studies have evaluated the addition of other drugs to sodium pentobarbital, such as lidocaine and phenytoin, and how such drugs affect the timing of events described elsewhere in this article.[43,44]

DEATH AS A PROCESS

Dying is well-understood to be a process, occurring over a time frame of months, hours, or minutes. Likewise, death is also a process that occurs over time. The cessation of cardiac function has been used to define the end of the process of dying and the beginning of the process of cellular death.[32] Once the heart has stopped, cellular death of the tissues of the body takes place over several hours to days. The term somatic death has been used to describe the cessation of cardiac and respiratory function. The term cell death refers to the biochemical cascade occurring after somatic death whereby cells are terminated via programmed cell death (apoptosis) or necrosis. Cell death can occur focally in the absence of complete somatic death, for example, in cases of acute injury. Somatic death can also occur independent of extensive cellular death, such as when a person is expediently revived after cardiopulmonary arrest. Despite this, these terms are useful in describing chronologically, which general physical processes we are referring to over time (**Fig. 3**).

The rate of cellular death varies based on the tissue in question. Established time frames guide transplant medicine as to best practices in organ procurement and

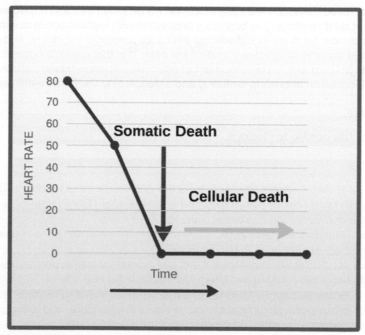

Fig. 3. Death over time.

transplantation.[45] A decrease in core body temperature can prolong the process of cellular death. Hypothermia treatments have been shown to have cytoprotective effects, in particular on nervous tissue.[46,47] This finding is of great interest and application for resuscitation science and critical care, with some hospitals routinely applying hypothermia treatment after cardiopulmonary resuscitation. The mechanisms of cellular death have been studied in human medicine extensively, with great focus on nervous tissue. Mitigating the consequences or forestalling the process of cellular death has significant implications for patients who experience cardiac arrest or neurologic trauma, or suffer from a stroke. Understanding biochemical processes such as excitotoxicity in this context, are critical and extensive research in this area reflects this.[48–50] The explanation of and criteria for brain death is beyond the scope of this article; however, controversy exists on criteria for this designation and thus variation in medical policies exists at this time.[51–55] Understanding the function and resilience of nervous tissue in the face of ischemia, hypoxia, and infarct over time has far-reaching consequences. Technological biomedical innovation and advanced scientific knowledge will have future moral, ethical, and societal ramifications in the areas of critical and end of life care. Progress in medicine and science will likely affect the fields of both veterinary and human medicine in ways that are difficult to anticipate. Research and advanced clinical interventions in end-of-life care and emergency medicine will guide practitioners in the future.

SUMMARY

This article attempted to incorporate and apply what is known about basic principles of acute death in human medicine to specific disease processes in veterinary patients. Much has yet to be understood regarding how veterinary patients die, without the intervention of euthanasia. Veterinary medicine will be influenced and impacted by the concepts of death and dying as biological processes with implications in several areas of social science. Such areas include the ethics, psychology, sociology, and cultural and spiritual aspects of veterinary end-of-life care. It is this author's hope that such knowledge will help with the development of effective, evidence-based palliative interventions focused on alleviating suffering and safeguarding the human–animal bond.

DISCLOSURE

The author has nothing to disclose.

REFERENCES

1. Bardale R. Ante mortem changes. In: Strub CG, Frederick LG, editors. The principles and practices of embalming. 3rd edition. Dallas (TX): Professional training schools and Robertine Frederick; 1989. p. 77–99.
2. Motta L, Mandara MT, Skerritt GC. Canine and feline intracranial meningiomas: an updated review. Vet J 2012;192(2):153–65.
3. Snyder JM, Shofer FS, Van Winkle TJ, et al. Canine intracranial primary neoplasia: 173 cases (1986-2003). J Vet Intern Med 2006;20(3):669–75.
4. Gitto L, Bolino G, Cina SJ. Sudden unexpected deaths due to intracranial meningioma: presentation of six fatal cases, review of the literature, and a discussion of the mechanisms of death. J Forensic Sci 2018;63(3):947–53.
5. Gurkanlar D, Er U, Sanli M, et al. Peritumoral brain edema in intracranial meningiomas. J Clin Neurosci 2005;12:750–3.
6. Smith ER, Madsen JR. Cerebral pathophysiology and critical care neurology: basic hemodynamic principles, cerebral perfusion and intracranial pressure. Semin Pediatr Neurol 2004;11(2):89–104.
7. Reeves A, Swenson R. Depression of consciousness. In: Disorders of the nervous system. Dartmouth Medical School; 2004. Available at: http://www.dartmouth.edu/~dons/part_2/chapter_17.html#chpt_17_summary. Accessed April 13, 2019.
8. Silva J, Chamadoira C, Cerejo A, et al. Clival meningioma presenting with respiratory arrest. Acta Neurochir (Wien) 2011;153(7):1509–10.
9. Turillazzi E, Bello S, Neri M, et al. Colloid cyst of the third ventricle, hypothalamus and heart: a dangerous link for sudden death. Diagn Pathol 2012;7(44):1–5.
10. Karli P, Gorgas D, Oevermann A, et al. Extracranial expansion of a feline meningioma. J Feline Med Surg 2013;15(8):749–53.
11. Matsuoka G, Eguchi BR, Tominaga T, et al. Treatment strategy for recurrent hemorrhage from meningioma: case report and literature review. World J Neurol 2018; 124:75–80.
12. Martin-Vaquero P, da Costa RC, Aeffner F, et al. Imaging diagnosis-hemorrhagic meningioma. Vet Radiol Ultrasound 2010;51(2):165–7.
13. Mandara MT, Reginato A, Foiani G, et al. Papillary meningioma in the dog: a clinicopathological case series. Res Vet Sci 2015;100:213–9.
14. Tomek A, Cizinauskas S, Doherr M, et al. Intracranial neoplasia in 61 cats: localization, tumour types and seizure patterns. J Feline Med Surg 2006;8:243–53.
15. Vischer AS, Connolly DJ, Coats CJ, et al. Arrhythmogenic right ventricular cardiomyopathy in boxer dogs: the diagnosis as a link to the human disease. Acta Myol 2017;36:135–50.
16. Basso C, Fox PR, Meurs KM, et al. Arrhythmogenic right ventricular cardiomyopathy causing sudden cardiac death in boxer dogs. Circulation 2004;109:1180–5.

17. Patil K, Halperin HR, Becker LB. Cardiac arrest: resuscitation and reperfusion. Circ Res 2018;116(12):2041–9.

18. Weisfeldt ML. A three phase temporal model for cardiopulmonary resuscitation following cardiac arrest. Trans Am Clin Climatol Assoc 2004;115:115–22.

19. Ewy GA. Cardiocerebral resuscitation, defibrillation and cardioversion. In: Jeremias A, Brown DL, editors. Cardiac intensive care. 2nd edition. Philadelphia: Saunders Elsevier; 2010. p. 652–72.

20. Goyal V, Jassal DS, Dhalla NS. Pathophysiology and prevention of sudden cardiac death. Can J Physiol Pharmacol 2016;94:237–44.

21. Hamzaoui O, Monnet X, Teboul JL. Pulsus paradoxus. Eur Respir J 2013;42(6):1696–705.

22. Reddy PS, Curtiss EL. Cardiac tamponade. Cardiol Clin 1990;8(4):627–37.

23. Ware WA, Hopper DL. Cardiac tumors in dogs: 1982–1995. J Vet Intern Med 1999;13:95–103.

24. Treggiari E, Pedro B, Dukes-McEwan J, et al. A descriptive review of cardiac tumors in dogs and cats. Vet Comp Oncol 2017;15(2):273–88.

25. Myerburg RJ. Sudden cardiac death: interface between pathophysiology and epidemiology. Card Electrophysiol Clin 2017;9(4):515–24.

26. Ristagno G, Tang W, Sun S, et al. Spontaneous gasping produces carotid blood flow during untreated cardiac arrest. Resuscitation 2007;75(2):366–71.

27. Wilkie LJ, Smith K, Fuentes VL. Cardiac pathology findings in 252 cats presented for necropsy; a comparison of cats with unexpected death versus other deaths. J Vet Cardiol 2015;17:S329–40.

28. McFadden ER, Warren EL. Observations on asthma mortality. Ann Intern Med 1997;127(2):142–7.

29. Rosenberg HF, Druey KM. Modeling asthma: pitfalls, promises and the road ahead. J Leukoc Biol 2018;104.41–8.

30. Venema C, Patterson C. Feline asthma: what's new and where might clinical practice be heading? J Feline Med Surg 2010;12:681–92.

31. Nogues MA, Benarroch E. Abnormalities of respiratory control and the respiratory motor unit. Neurologist 2008;14(5):273–88.

32. Parnia S. Erasing death. 1st edition. New York: HarperCollins e-books; 2013.

33. Lisowska-Myjak B. Uremic toxins and their effects on multiple organ systems. Nephron Clin Pract 2014;128:303–11.

34. Dastani M. Coronary artery disease in patients with chronic kidney disease: a brief literature review. Rev Clin Med 2015;2(4):178–82.

35. Pouchelon JL, Atkins CE, Bussadori MA, et al. Cardiovascular–renal axis disorders in the domestic dog and cat: a veterinary consensus statement. J Small Anim Pract 2015;56:537–52.

36. Kennedy JS. The pathophysiology of hypovolemia and dehydration. J AHIMA 2006;77(7):78–80.

37. Pellegrino FC. Renal-associated encephalopathy: bibliographic review. An Vet Murcia 2009;25:47–57.

38. Edwards DF, Legendre AM, McCracken MD. Hypoglycemia and chronic renal failure in the cat. J Am Vet Med Assoc 1987;190(4):435–6.

39. Gu ZZ. Effects of hyperoxia and hypoxia on cerebral circulation and intracranial pressure. Sheng Li Xue Bao 1993;45(5):415–22.

40. Crellin SJ, Katz KD. Pentobarbital toxicity after self-administration of euthasol veterinary euthanasia medication. Case Rep Emerg Med 2016;2016:6270491.

41. American Society of Heathy System Pharmacists. AHFS drug information. Bethesda (MD): 2009. p. 2577–99. Available at: https://www.pharmacompass.com/chemistry-chemical-name/phenobarbital. Accessed January 15, 2020.

42. Tameem A, Krovvidi H. Cerebral physiology. Br J Anaesth 2013;13(4):113–8.

43. FDA/CVM FOIA NADA-119-807-Beuthanasia D-Obtained 11/2/17. Available at: https://www.fda.gov/AnimalVeterinary/Products/ApprovedAnimalDrugProducts/ucm2006466.htm. Accessed February 27, 2019.

44. Evans AT, Broadstone R, Stapleton J, et al. Comparison of pentobarbital alone and pentobarbital in combination with lidocaine for euthanasia in dogs. J Am Vet Med Assoc 1993;203(5):664–6.

45. Bernat JL, D' Alessandro AM, Port FK, et al. Report of a national conference on donation after cardiac death. Am J Transplant 2006;6(2):281–91.

46. Jackson TC, Kochnek PM. A new vision for therapeutic hypothermia in the era of targeted temperature management: a speculative synthesis. Ther Hypothermia Temp Manag 2019;9(1):13–47.

47. Arrocj J, Holzer M, Havel C, et al. Hypothermia for neuroprotection in adults after cardiopulmonary resuscitation. Cochrane Database Syst Rev 2016;(2):CD004128.

48. Woitzik J, Pinczolitis A, Hecht N, et al. Excitotoxicity and metabolic changes in association with infarct progression. Stroke 2014;45:1183–5.

49. Weita T, Zhang S, Wang YT. Excitotoxicity and stroke: identifying novel targets for neuroprotection. Prog Neurobiol 2014;115:157–88.

50. Tehse J, Taghibiglou C. The overlooked aspect of excitotoxity: glutamate-independent excitotoxicity in traumatic brain injuries. Eur J Neurosci 2019; 49(9):1157–70.

51. Rady MY, Verheijde JL. Neuroscience and awareness in the dying brain: implications for organ donation practices. J Crit Care 2016;34:121–3.

52. Parnia S, Spearpoint K, de Vos G. AWARE -AWAreness during REsuscitation- a prospective study. Resuscitation 2014;85:1799–805.

53. Reid VL, McDonald R, Nwosu AC, et al. A systemically structured review of biomarkers of dying in cancer patients in the last months of life; an exploration of the biology of dying. PLoS One 2017;12(4):e0175123.

54. Reagan EM, Nguyen RT, Ravishankar ST, et al. Monitoring the relationship between changes in cerebral oxygenation and electroencephalography patterns during cardiopulmonary resuscitation: a feasibility study. Crit Care Med 2018; 46(5):757–63.

55. Parnia S, Yang J, Nguyen R, et al. Cerebral oximetry during cardiac arrest. A multicenter study of neurologic outcomes and survival. Crit Care Med 2016; 44(9):1663–74.

Pharmacologic Methods
An Update on Optimal Presedation and Euthanasia Solution Administration

Sheilah A. Robertson, BVMS (Hons), PhD

KEYWORDS

- Sedation • Anesthesia • Pre-euthanasia • Euthanasia • Adverse events • Route
- Injection

KEY POINTS

- Sedation or anesthesia prior to euthanasia improves the experience for the pet and owner. Anesthesia is required if a nonintravenous route is used for euthanasia.
- Some sedative and anesthetic drugs can be given by the oral, oral transmucosal, and buccal routes to avoid intramuscular or subcutaneous injections.
- The ideal pre-euthanasia sedation protocol for each individual patient remains elusive but new information from preanesthetic studies can be applied.
- In the era of drug shortages, clinicians should be familiar with several techniques for sedation and euthanasia.

 Video content accompanies this article at http://www.vetsmall.theclinics.com

INTRODUCTION

Life is meaningful because it is a story. Both a story and a life depend crucially on how it ends. In stories, endings matter.
—Atul Gawande, Being Mortal: Medicine and What Matters in the End

Performing euthanasia is an important part of veterinary practice and should be a day 1 competency skill for veterinarians. A veterinarians' primary responsibility is to cause minimal stress or pain to the animal during the procedure. Euthanasia involves other stakeholders, however, which, depending on the context and setting, may involve veterinary nurses, technicians and other clinic staff, lay personnel, shelter personnel, research personnel, children, owners, and other caregivers. The potential psychological and emotional impacts on these people must not be underestimated, and these do not end after an animal's death.

Lap of Love Veterinary Hospice Inc., 17804 N US Highway, Lutz, FL, 33549, USA
E-mail address: drrobertson@lapoflove.com

Vet Clin Small Anim 50 (2020) 525–543
https://doi.org/10.1016/j.cvsm.2019.12.004
0195-5616/20/© 2019 Elsevier Inc. All rights reserved.

Performing a perfect euthanasia may be a lofty goal, but it should be what veterinarians strive for every time; despite how often this procedure is performed, there is a surprising lack of published data on best practices based on well-conducted research or clinical studies.[1] The number of professionals involved in end-of-life veterinary care, palliative care, and in-home euthanasia services is expanding globally and, with the creation of professional organizations dedicated to education and research in these specialties, it is predicted that helpful information will be collected and disseminated. Tamara Shearer's article, "Standardization of Data Collection to Document Adverse Events Associated with Euthanasia," in this issue discusses standardization of data collection to document adverse events associated with euthanasia; this will be invaluable for moving forward.

Meanwhile the current literature should be reviewed for potential protocols that deserve more investigation and data looked for on successful preanesthetic protocols that can be used in the euthanasia setting.

UNDESIRABLE SIDE-EFFECTS

The undesirable effects of pre-euthanasia sedation and euthanasia include, but are not limited to, reactions to injection(s), dysphoria, excitation, vocalization, vomiting, muscle activity, and agonal breaths.[1] Some of these occur when the animal is still aware (eg, at the time of injection and during the onset of sedation or anesthesia) and may cause distress, and, even if animals are unconscious at the time of these events (eg, agonal breaths), they are certainly unpleasant for observers.

WHY SEDATE OR ANESTHETIZE BEFORE EUTHANASIA?

Intravenous (IV) administration of pentobarbital and pentobarbital combinations (eg, pentobarbital plus phenytoin) is an acceptable euthanasia method for companion animals.[2] Physical restraint is stressful for many animals and requires skilled personnel, ideally trained in low stress handling; if incorrectly performed, the animal or handler may be injured. Performing venipuncture or placing an IV catheter to administer euthanasia drugs also requires skill. For the benefit of all stakeholders, pre-euthanasia sedation is strongly recommended; therefore, euthanasia is a 2-step process (**Box 1**).

The benefits of sedation for the animal and involved personnel generally are accepted as greatly outweighing any potential negative effects. Adopting pre-euthanasia sedation (or anesthesia protocols), however, requires additional record keeping and added expense. Using a 2-step process may add time but also can

---

Box 1
Advantages of pre-euthanasia sedation or anesthesia

- Allows owners to see their pet relaxed and peaceful
- May improve an owner's experience
- Allows for minimal restraint during euthanasia
- Increases the choice of euthanasia techniques (eg, when IV injection is not possible)
- Increases safety during the euthanasia process
- May decrease the negative emotional impact that performing euthanasia can have on personnel
- May decrease unwanted side effects during euthanasia and immediately postmortem

reduce the time taken for successful euthanasia when working with large dogs or difficult to manage dogs or cats. This additional step may itself result in adverse events, can be unpredictable, and can affect the euthanasia process. This is why gathering information on what is an ideal protocol is needed (**Box 2**).

PRE-EUTHANASIA SEDATION AND ANESTHESIA

The difference between sedation, anesthesia, and unconsciousness is critically important; the American Veterinary Medical Association Guidelines for the Euthanasia of Animals: 2020 edition, clearly state, "placement of intraosseous catheters for administration of euthanasia agents and intracardiac, intrahepatic, intrasplenic, or intrarenal injections are acceptable only when performed on anesthetized or unconscious animals (with the exception of intrahepatic injections in cats)."[2] This means that if the first step is omitted but IV access is not successfully achieved, starting again and sedating or anesthetizing the patients before proceeding with a practical alternative route for administration of euthanasia drugs required. These alternative routes are discussed in Kathleen Cooney's article, "Common and Alternative Routes of Euthanasia Solution Administration," in this issue.

Definitions

The following definitions are taken from a textbook of veterinary anesthesia.[3] *Sedation* is defined as a state characterized by central depression accompanied by drowsiness (**Box 3**). The patient generally is unaware of its surroundings but can become aroused and is responsive to noxious stimulation. *Tranquillization* is often used interchangeably with sedation but is different; it results in a behavioral change: anxiety is relieved and the animal is relaxed but remains aware of its surroundings. *Anesthesia*, in the context of this article, means general anesthesia; this is a drug-induced unconsciousness characterized by depression of the central nervous system; the patient is not arousable by noxious stimuli. Performing a toe pinch, which elicits no withdrawal, can be used for confirmation and this can be done under a blanket out of an owner's view.

To avoid confusion, correctly defining routes of administration is important, especially when the terms oral, oral transmucosal (OTM), and buccal, are used. In this text, oral means that the drug is swallowed and usually this is a tablet or capsule formulation; OTM means that a drug was placed in contact with oral mucosa, which may include the sublingual area or the cheek pouch; buccal means the liquid drug or gel was placed specifically into the cheek pouch.

Oral Administration

Gabapentin
The exact mechanism of action of gabapentin has not been fully elucidated but it was first developed as an antiepileptic agent. It has a suitable pharmacokinetic profile for

---

Box 2
The ideal pre-euthanasia sedation protocol

- Reliable—produces similar results in a wide variety of patients
- Predictable—produces the desired effect within a predictable time and for a predicable duration
- Versatile—can be given IM, SC, orally, or by the OTM route
- Devoid of unwanted side effects

> **Box 3**
> **Definitions related to the state of consciousness**
>
> Sedation: central depression accompanied by drowsiness. The patient can be aroused and is responsive to noxious stimulation.
>
> Tranquillization: a behavioral change in which anxiety is relieved, and the animal is relaxed but remains aware of its surroundings
>
> General anesthesia: a drug-induced unconsciousness. The patient is not arousable by noxious stimuli.

oral administration in cats, with a reported mean systemic availability close to 89% in 1 study and a median bioavailability of almost 95% in another.[4,5] It frequently is used to decreases stress and anxiety caused by transport and veterinary visits in cats.[6] Gabapentin reduced fear responses in cage-trapped community cats.[7] These reports support its use in cats when a euthanasia appointment is scheduled for a known time; it has no strong or aversive flavor or smell and cats that are still voluntarily eating usually consume it in a small amount of wet food. It also can be formulated as a suspension and given by syringe.[7] Transdermal gabapentin is not effective.[5] Time to maximum plasma concentration and peak clinical effects is between 1 hour and 2 hours.[4,5,7] Doses are usually given as milligrams per cat, most often 50 mg, 100 mg, or 150 mg. In published studies, the effective doses on a milligrams/kilogram basis range from 10 to 29.4.[5,6] The effects of oral gabapentin often include a very sedated, or sleepy, cat (Video 1). In the United States, gabapentin is a controlled drug (Schedule IV) in some states.

Melatonin

Based on the success of melatonin for reducing anxiety in pediatric patients, its value as a calming agent in dogs has been assessed.[8,9] Dogs given 5 mg/kg of melatonin were scored as calmer 90 minutes to 2 hours after administration and in some dogs the dose of propofol required for anesthesia induction was reduced.[9] In this study, dogs were not aggressive; however, melatonin is used as part of the chill protocol to manage aggressive and fearful dogs (discussed later).[10]

Trazodone

Trazodone in a 5-hydroxytryptamine antagonist and reuptake inhibitor. It is reported to decrease transport and examination related stress in cats[11,12] and alleviate stress in hospitalized dogs.[13]

In cats, a single dose of oral trazodone (50 mg/cat or 100 mg/cat) caused sedation and decreased the signs of anxiety related to being examined; cats looked sleepy, which may be beneficial for owners.[11,12] Behavioral changes occur within 30 minutes of administration but peak at approximately 2 hours. When adjusted for body weight, the reported doses are 50 mg/cat = 7.7 mg/kg to 16.7 mg/kg and 100 mg/cat = 21 mg/kg to 33.3 mg/kg[11,12]; 100 mg/cat given 2 hours prior to a euthanasia appointment is recommended—this applies to in-home euthanasia and for cats being transported to a clinic.

In dogs, individual variation in response to administration is common and not surprising based on a pharmacokinetic study in which time to peak plasma concentration and oral bioavailability were highly variable even in a group of purpose-bred beagles.[14] Suggested doses range from 4 mg/kg to 12 mg/kg.[13–15] For these reasons, test doses are suggested to assess the individual patient response; this may be possible with a planned canine euthanasia, but trazodone alone should not be relied on to facilitate handling in other settings. When used, suggested doses range from 4 mg/kg to 12 mg/kg. Drugs and doses for oral sedation of dogs and cats are shown in **Table 1**.

Pentobarbital

Pentobarbital (powdered formulation) alone (63.2 mg/kg ± 5.1 mg/kg) in capsules placed into food resulted in lateral recumbency in 6 of 7 dogs in a mean time of 59 minutes.[16] In the 21 years since that study, to this author's knowledge, no other studies using this method have been published. It is, however, frequently mentioned and discussed.[17] Smith[17] suggests using the powdered formulation of pentobarbital but has used the liquid form and products containing pentobarbital and phenytoin. Because of the bitter taste, gel capsules should be used; unfortunately, the liquid formulations can cause these to melt or leak, so they should be prepared close to the time they are needed. When using the powdered formulation of pentobarbital, 1 g per 11.5 kg has been suggested and the dog should be left undisturbed for 45 minutes to 90 minutes for the drug to take effect.[17] This dose is approximately 90 mg/kg, which is similar to recommended IV dose; therefore, if possible, aim to administer 2 times to 3 times this amount to hasten onset of action and to enhance the depth of sedation or anesthesia. Regardless of which formulation is used, a capsule machine (eg, The Capsule Machine, Capsule Connection, Prescott, Arizona) is highly recommended for filling gel capsules.

A combination of encapsulated tiletamine-zolazepam and acepromazine (approximately 20 mg/kg and 2 mg/kg, respectively) placed in food has been used to sedate free-roaming dogs and dogs prior to euthanasia. Success rates (capture or lateral recumbency) were 63% to 87%, respectively, within a time frame of under 50 minutes.[16,18]

ORAL TRANSMUCOSAL OR BUCCAL ROUTES

The OTM and buccal routes of administration are used for administration of drugs that have poor oral bioavailability due to hepatic metabolism, prior to reaching the systemic circulation (first-pass effect) (**Table 2**). Owners can be taught to use this route, and it avoids the need to inject a patient. The drugs should be in a liquid or gel formulation and, ideally, are deposited under the tongue or into the cheek pouch. They should be given slowly enough or in a sufficiently small volume to avoid the drug being swallowed. In fractious animals, the drug can be squirted into the mouth or given after a muzzle is placed. A nylon or basked muzzle still allows access to the oral cavity.

Acepromazine is a sedative with authorization for use in dogs and cats. Oral bioavailability in dogs is low (approximately 20%)[19]; therefore, the OTM or buccal route is used to avoid the first-pass effect, and, although there are no published

Table 1
Recommended drugs for oral sedation in dogs and cats; doses are given as milligrams/ kilogram

Drug	Dog	Cat
Gabapentin	10.0–20.0	10.0–30.0
Melatonin[a]	5.0	Not reported but same dose as for dog is suggested
Trazodone	4.0–12.0	8.0–33.0

[a] This dose is suggested if melatonin alone is being used. In dogs, the chill protocol (see **Table 3** and text for details) suggests lower doses.

Table 2
Drugs for oral transmucosal and buccal sedation in dogs and cats

Drug	Dog	Cat	Comments
Acepromazine	0.025–0.05 mg/kg	0.05–0.1 mg/kg	Dogs: also used as a component of the chill protocol; see text and **Table 3** for details. Not well documented in cats, but higher doses are recommended in cats compared with dogs.
Buprenorphine	Not practical Requires high doses (volumes) and salivation is reported.	0.03–0.03 mg/kg	Highly recommended in painful cats. Allow 30–45 min for an effect; sedation is minimal.
Dexmedetomidine	0.02–0.033 mg/kg	Not recommended	
Detomidine[a]	0.5–1.0 mg/m^2 The 1.0-mg/m^2 dose is approximately 0.037 mg/kg or 37 μg/kg.	Not recommended	Dosed on body surface area See text for details.
Tiletamine-zolazepam	This route is not well documented in dogs.	5.0 mg/kg	7.5 mg/kg is associated with salivation.

[a] Equine oromucosal gel formulation.

data on bioavailability when given this way, clinical experience suggests it is effective and it is a component of the chill protocol (discussed later).[12]

Buprenorphine is an effective OTM analgesic and can be a valuable adjunct to the pre-euthanasia protocol, especially in painful cats. When the IV route is not easily accessible and intramuscular (IM) routes are best avoided (eg, skinny patients), it is a good choice, because the subcutaneous (SC) route is ineffective. It is unlikely, however, to provide good sedation.[20–23] It is well accepted by most cats and recommended doses are 0.02 mg/kg to 0.03 mg/kg. It has less utility in dogs because higher doses (volumes) are required due to lower bioavailability and salivation is reported.[24]

α₂-Adrenergic Agonist Agents

Dexmedetomidine provides reliable dose-related sedation in dogs and cats and has the benefit of providing analgesia and muscle relaxation. α₂-Adrenergic agonist agents commonly are used as a component of an injectable pre-euthanasia sedation or anesthetic protocol. Although effective sedation was achieved with dexmedetomidine alone or in combination with buprenorphine when given by the OTM route in cats, it cannot be recommended because of the high incidence of vomiting and salivation.[25,26]

In dogs, OTM administration of dexmedetomidine can produce profound sedation at doses ranging from 0.02 mg/kg to 0.033 mg/kg with a low incidence of ptyalism and vomiting.[27,28] Cohen and Bennett[27] described this technique in 4 aggressive dogs. In 1 case, the drug was deposited into the conjunctival sac when the dog lunged and resulted in good sedation; in other cases, buccal administration was possible through a basket muzzle.

Detomidine is available in an oromucosal gel formulation for horses (Dormosedan gel [detomidine hydrochloride], 7.6 mg/mL [Zoetis, Parsippany, NJ]). It has been used in dogs to produce sedation and facilitate handling and for minor procedures (eg, clipping and placement of a jugular catheter).[29,30] The gel is administered into the buccal cavity using a microsyringe after transferring it from the product's dosing syringe; wearing gloves or a finger cot is advised. A dose of 0.35 mg/m^2 (approximately 0.012–0.016 mg/kg) resulted in good sedation, decreased anxiety, and increased ease of handling; onset of effect was noticeable within 15 minutes of treatment and peaked at 45 minutes.[30] No vomiting or salivation was noted; bradycardia was reported but is expected with this class of drug.[29] Messenger and colleagues[29] used 0.5 mg/m^2 to place jugular catheters in dogs; for conversion of square meters to milligrams/kilogram, see the *Merck Veterinary Manual*.[31] These studies were performed in a small population (n = 6) of healthy institute-owned animals; however, anecdotal reports of its use for pre-euthanasia sedation in dogs with a wide variety of temperaments and health status are positive, with many practitioners using higher than published doses. If the practitioner or owner cannot place the gel into the buccal pouch or oral cavity, it can be mixed with peanut butter or thick syrup and placed on a plastic plate or smeared on a favorite toy for the dog to lick. A dose of 1.0 mg/m^2 (approximately 0.037 mg/kg [37 µg/kg]) produced lateral recumbency in approximately 40 minutes[29]; therefore, this is a suggested starting dose for pre-euthanasia sedation. The volume of detomidine gel is approximately 0.005 mL/kg; therefore, 0.1 mL is administered to 20-kg dog.

Tiletamine-zolazepam is efficacious by the buccal route in cats (discussed later) but is not available in all countries. Alternatives, such as detomidine (0.5 mg/kg of the injectable equine solution [10 mg/mL]) and ketamine (10 mg/kg) produce reliable sedation in cats within 10 minutes to 25 minutes, but the side effects of vomiting and salivation are unacceptable.[32]

Dogs and cats may look extremely sedate and often are recumbent after administration of α_2-adrenergic agonist drugs (by any route), but they are arousable, especially by loud noises or sudden noxious stimuli, and this can happen quickly and be unexpected, so it is important to be proceed cautiously to prevent injury to anyone close to the patient. If the patient responds, more sedation (with other drugs) or anesthesia may be needed. Even high doses of this class of drug do not produce general anesthesia, so only IV administration of euthanasia is appropriate.

Dissociative Anesthetic Agents

The combination of a dissociative agent and a benzodiazepine (tiletamine-zolazepam) is a widely used IM anesthetic in dogs and cats. One of its major drawbacks is that it frequently causes a reaction, such as vocalization and movement, when injected, which is thought to be a result of its low pH (2–3.5). In cats, the buccal route of administration is an alternative to consider.[33]

The effects of 2 doses administered into the cheek pouch of cats have been reported: 5 mg/kg (= 0.1 mL/kg) and 7.5 mg/kg (= 0.15 mL/kg). Neither dose produced retching or vomiting; ptyalism did not occur after the 5-mg/kg dose but was reported in 3 of the 7 cats after the higher dose—this was not statistically different but is clinically relevant.[33] Posture, the response to clippers, and physical restraint were recorded over time, with no differences noted between doses. Within 15 minutes, most cats were laterally recumbent (but some could raise their head), did not respond to clippers being turned on, and did not resist physical restraint. A dose of 5 mg/kg is suggested to avoid hypersalivation; the absence of response to a noxious stimulation must be confirmed if a non-IV site is chosen for administration of euthanasia solution.

Ketamine should not be used alone for immobilization in dogs or cats because it results in rigidity and salivation and is unpleasant for the patient and observers.

INTRANASAL ADMINISTRATION

Intranasal (IN) administration of medetomidine and dexmedetomidine have been compared with the IM route in dogs.[34,35] Dexmedetomidine, 0.02 mg/kg, was administered IN using a mucosal atomization device attached to a Luer lock syringe, with equal volumes administered into each nostril while holding the dog's head up at a 30° angle or injected into the rectus femoris muscle.[34] Onset of action and time to peak sedation were not significantly different between routes (onset time: means of 6.3 min and 9.4 min and peak effect: 23.5 min and 28.0 min for IN and IM, respectively). Sedations scores were higher in the IN group mean of 10 out of a possible score of 14, compared with the IM group (mean of 6), but there was variability in both groups. No adverse events were reported. IN drops, IN atomization, and IM injection of medetomidine (0.04 mg/kg) were compared in 18 dogs (n = 6 in each group).[35] Ease of administration was not different with each technique. Onset and degree of sedation were similar in the IN atomization and IM groups (onset times of 7.2 min ± 2.5 min and 6.3 min ± 2.0 min, respectively). IN drops were much less effective with a slower onset time (20.7 min ± 5.4 min) and lower sedation scores achieved. IN administration is an alternative noninvasive route of administration for medetomidine and dexmedetomidine in dogs, but an atomizer should be used.[34,35]

THE CHILL PROTOCOL

The chill protocol combines gabapentin, melatonin, and acepromazine and is recommended to facilitate interactions with aggressive and fearful dogs.[10] It is a 3-step process (Fig. 1, Table 3). All 3 drugs can be administered by the owner, but this protocol requires planning and the shortest lead time needed for it to work is 2 hours (if the first dose of gabapentin is omitted). This protocol was developed to facilitate care of aggressive and fearful dogs in a clinical setting; in a pre-euthanasia setting, higher doses of drugs can be used.

SYSTEMIC ADMINISTRATION
Intramuscular and Subcutaneous Routes—Cats

Many clinicians choose to use an anesthetic premedication protocol that they are comfortable and familiar with as their pre-euthanasia sedation. This requires no ordering of extra drugs and is encouraged because it means they know what to expect (eg, onset time, reaction to injection, and depth of sedation) and have likely already seen and dealt with unwanted side effects. If dexmedetomidine is a component of the sedation protocol, adding ondansetron (0.22 mg/kg IM) is highly recommended to prevent vomiting.[36] A premedication (sedation or tranquillization) technique is suitable if euthanasia drugs are administered IV. In cats, many people choose one of the many so-called kitty magic drug combinations that contain an analgesic (eg, butorphanol), anesthetic (usually a dissociative), and α₂-adrenergic agent (eg, dexmedetomidine) to provide general anesthesia so that non-IV routes can be used for euthanasia.

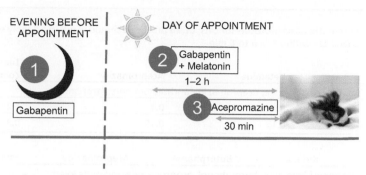

Fig. 1. The 3 drugs and 3 steps included in the chill protocol for fearful and aggressive dogs.

Total IM anesthesia can be achieved with a single injection when tiletamine-zolazepam, dexmedetomidine, and butorphanol are combined[37]; however, tiletamine-zolazepam is not available in all countries. Other popular combinations are ketamine, dexmedetomidine, and an opioid, often butorphanol.[38] Some clinicians use midazolam to increase muscle relaxation; for example, Polson and colleagues[39] used a combination of midazolam, medetomidine, ketamine, and butorphanol or buprenorphine to anesthetize female cats and this has become known as the cat or kitten quad technique. All these protocols are suitable for pre-euthanasia anesthesia.

A combination of tiletamine-zolazepam, ketamine, and xylazine (TKX) has been used successfully as an IM anesthesia induction protocol in community cats, with the advantage that a total volume of 0.27 mL ± 0.09 mL (mean ± SD) is sufficient for most cats and it has a rapid onset of action (<5 minutes).[40] The mixture is made by reconstituting powdered tiletamine-zolazepam with 4 mL of ketamine (100 mg/mL) and 1 mL of xylazine (100 mg/mL), resulting in each milliliter of reconstituted TKX contained 50 mg of tiletamine, 50 mg of zolazepam, 80 mg of ketamine, and 20 mg of xylazine. Other protocols have been developed that are suitable for IM and SC administration and to minimize the volume of injection (**Table 4**).[41]

Table 3
Recommended doses and routes of administration for the canine chill protocol (reference)

Drug and Route of Administration	Time of Administration and Dose		
	Evening Before Appointment	1–2 h Before Appointment	30 min Before Appointment
Gabapentin PO	20–25 mg/kg	20–25 mg/kg	
Melatonin PO		Small dog 0.5–1.0 mg Medium dog 1.0–3.0 mg Large dog 5.0 mg	
Acepromazine OTM			0.025–0.05 mg/kg

Note: doses of melatonin are milligrams per dog based on size.
Lap of Love Resources[41]

Table 4
Suggested pre-euthanasia protocols for cats; these protocols should result in a deeply sedated or anesthetized cat within 3 min to 6 min

Weight (kg)	Ketamine	Acepromazine	Tiletamine-Zolazepam
1. A combination of ketamine, acepromazine and tiletamine-zolazepam			
≤4.5	0.1	0.1	0.2
4.5–9.0	0.15	0.15	0.3

Weight (kg)	Ketamine	Butorphanol	Acepromazine	Midazolam
2. A combination of ketamine, butorphanol, acepromazine and midazolam				
≤4.5	0.3	0.3	0.1	0.3
4.5–9.0	0.4	0.4	0.1	0.4

Weight (kg)	Dose (mL)
3. Using Tiletamine-Zolazepam Reconstituted with Acepromazine (2.5 mL) and Ketamine (2.5 mL)	
≤4.5	0.2
4.5–9.0	0.3

Weight (kg)	Dose (mL)
4. Using Tiletamine-Zolazepam Reconstituted with Acepromazine (5 mL)	
≤4.5	0.1
4.5–9.0	0.2

Drug concentrations: tiletamine-zolazepam = 100 mg/mL (50 mg/mL tiletamine + 50 mg/mL zolazepam); ketamine = 100 mg/mL; acepromazine = 10 mg/mL; midazolam = 5 mg/mL; and butorphanol 10 mg/mL.
Note: nalbuphine (not a controlled substance) can be substituted for butorphanol.
Doses given in milliliters; all drugs are combined in a single syringe prior to injection.
Route of administration: IM or SC.

Newer Drugs

Alfaxalone

Alfaxalone (Alfaxan Multidose, Jurox Animal Health, North Kansas City, MO) is a neurosteroid anesthetic and is approved for IV use in dogs and cats in the United Sates. In some countries, it has market authorization for IM use in cats and this route is gaining popularity, albeit extralabel, in North America. It has a pH of approximately 7[42] and is not an irritant to tissues, offering some advantages over the acidic dissociative agents.

Depending on the IM dose of alfaxalone given and the drugs it is combined with, anything from light sedation to general anesthesia sufficient for surgery can be achieved.[43–47] IM administration of alfaxalone (2 mg/kg) and butorphanol (0.2 mg/kg) produced no clinically significant differences in echocardiographic measurements to those measured in the same cats when conscious, making IV access more likely. Cats (n = 10) were laterally recumbent 7.5 minutes ± 3.8 (mean ± SD) after injection.[46] In a pilot study (n = 6) designed to evaluate a combination of IM alfaxalone (2–3 mg/kg) and butorphanol (0.4 mg/kg) for feline blood donation, all cats were adequately sedate for the procedure and achieved lateral recumbency in a median time of 11.5 minutes (range 6–20), and hypotension was not reported.[44] In another blood collection study, which recruited client owned cats, IM alfaxalone (2 mg/kg) and butorphanol (0.2 mg/kg) (group AB) were compared with dexmedetomidine (10 µg/kg) and butorphanol (0.2 mg/kg) (group DB) in a randomized crossover study.[45] There were no differences in sedation scores between the groups, but group AB had higher muscle relaxation scores. More cats in group DB became laterally recumbent, but there was no different in time to reach this posture. Blood collection with a 21G butterfly needle inserted in the jugular vein was successful in 7 of the 10 group AB cats and 8 of the 10 group DB cats. One cat in group DB vomited; 9 of the 10 cats tolerated both combinations of IM injections well, given a score of 0 of a maximum of 3. One cat became fractious during injection with both protocols. The investigators concluded that alfaxalone was a suitable alternative to dexmedetomidine but noted that neither protocol was 100% reliable.[45] Video 2 is of a nonsedated cat being given 2 mg/kg of alfaxalone combined with 0.2 mg/kg of butorphanol in the dorsal epaxial muscles; a 25G needle was used, the cat was minimally restrained and the injection given slowly.

Higher doses of alfaxalone (5 mg/kg vs 2 mg/kg) combined with butorphanol provide better sedation; however, the volume of injection becomes an issue;[47] the current commercially available formulation is a 1% solution; therefore, 5 mg/kg equates to a volume of 0.5 mL/kg. A more concentrated formulation of alfaxalone would provide all the benefits (described previously) and avoid the need for large volumes of injectate. The use of a new formulation of 4% (40 mg/mL) alfaxalone has been described in bighorn sheep (Ovis canadensis), with the investigators stating that this concentration greatly increased the utility of the drug when volume is a limiting factor.[48]

Anesthesia sufficient for castration can be achieved with alfaxalone (3 mg/kg), dexmedetomidine (10 µg/kg), and butorphanol (0.2 mg/kg); and Khenissi and colleagues[43] concluded that alfaxalone was a suitable substitute for ketamine (5 mg/mL). In this study, they carefully recorded reaction to IM (lumbar muscles) placement of the needle (23G) and reaction to injection. Insertion of the needle evoked a minor reaction, but injection caused significant responses indicating pain, regardless of whether the injection contained alfaxalone or ketamine combined with dexmedetomidine and butorphanol. It is not possible to determine if the reactions were due to irritation—a so-called ketamine sting often is spoken about but not well documented—or volume, which is suspected to be the trigger with alfaxalone. In this study the volume of dexmedetomidine and butorphanol were constant, but alfaxalone at 3 mg/kg is 0.3 mL/kg compared with 0.05 mL/kg when ketamine is dosed at 5 mg/kg.[43]

Subcutaneous administration of alfaxalone
There is 1 report of SC administration of alfaxalone (3 mg/kg) and butorphanol (0.2 mg/kg) in hyperthyroid cats; time to maximum sedation varied between 30 minutes and 45 minutes.[49] Although the sedation scores were quite variable, the goal of the study (to administer iodine-131 with minimal restraint) was achievable in all 20 cats at 45 minutes.[49] In this study, 56% of cats flinched or vocalized during injection and in 24% tremors were noted during treatment and were related to noise and handling. As with all euthanasia appointments, the veterinary care staff should remain quiet, avoid sudden noises (eg, silence phones), touch patents gently and slowly, and if possible not move them after they are sedated.

INTRAMUSCULAR AND SUBCUTANEOUS ROUTES—DOGS

As with cats, many clinicians use a protocol they would use for sedation prior to anesthesia, but usually choose to give higher doses. Many suitable protocols that utilize tiletamine-zolazepam, dexmedetomidine, and butorphanol are in available in open-access journal articles.[37] In countries where tiletamine-zolazepam is not

Table 5
Suggested pre-euthanasia sedation protocol for dogs; this protocol should result in a deeply sedated or anesthetized dog within 3 min to 6 min

A Quick Reference Guide (Milliliters of Each Drug) for Specific Weight Ranges				
Weight (kg)	Ketamine	Xylazine	Butorphanol	Acepromazine
0–9	0.3	0.1	0.2	0.1
9.5–18	0.6	0.2	0.4	0.2
19–27	0.9	0.3	0.6	0.3
28–36	1.2	0.4	0.8	0.4
37–45	1.5	0.5	1.0	0.5
46–55	1.8	0.6	1.2	0.6

Drug concentrations: ketamine = 100 mg/mL; acepromazine = 10 mg/mL; xylazine 100 mg/mL; and butorphanol 10 mg/mL.
Note: nalbuphine (not a controlled substance) can be substituted for butorphanol.
Route of administration: IM or SC.
Dose: ketamine, 3.3 mg/kg; xylazine, 1.1 mg/kg; butorphanol, 0.22 mg/kg; and acepromazine, 0.11 mg/kg. Drugs are combined in a single syringe.

available, other reliable combinations include ketamine, xylazine, butorphanol, and acepromazine (**Table 5**).[41]

IM administration of alfaxalone is reported in dogs.[50–52] Dose-dependent anesthetic effects with minimal cardiovascular and respiratory depression were noted with IM alfaxalone at 5.0 mg/kg, 7.5 mg/kg, and 10 mg/kg; all dogs given the 2 higher doses could be orotracheally intubated within approximately 8 minutes to 10 minutes.[50] Time to lateral recumbency was similar with all 3 doses (mean time <4 minutes). If a maximum volume of 0.5 mL/kg is adhered to for an IM injection, the current commercially available 1% solution of alfaxalone is impractical, requiring more than 1 IM injection for doses greater than 5 mg/kg, and vocalizing and struggling were reported in some dogs given a single 0.5-mL/kg injection.[50] To overcome the volume issue, lower doses (1 mg/kg, 2 mg/kg, and 4 mg/kg) of alfaxalone have been used to produce sedation rather than anesthesia in dogs.[50,51] Unfortunately, these sedative doses are accompanied by unacceptable side effects, especially strong reactions to noise. Lower doses combined with other sedatives or tranquillizers or the use of a more concentrated formulation of alfaxalone (eg, 4% [40 mg/mL]), may overcome many of these issues in the future.[48]

CLINICAL TIPS WHEN GIVING INTRAMUSCULAR INJECTIONS

Aversive reactions to IM injection are commonly reported in dogs and cats, regardless of the drug(s) used. Many factors may play a role, including the pH of the injectate, volume, size of the needle, speed of injection, and the injection site (**Fig. 2**). It is recommended to use the smallest size needle possible; choose the site and gently rub the area to see the patient's response (rubbing also may act as a distraction) and/or manipulate the sensory pathway from that site; if there is minimal to no reaction, insert the needle and pause. If there is still minimal response after needle insertion, inject slowly; slow expansion of the SC or IM tissue may be less painful. If the patient strongly reacts to the initial needle insertion, it is necessary to proceed immediately and inject quickly.

Another factor to consider is whether or not the patient has developed hypersensitivity. Dogs and cats with chronic painful conditions, such as osteoarthritis or

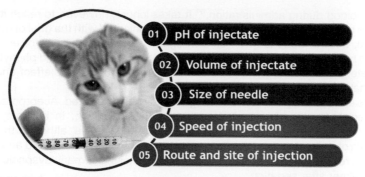

01 pH of injectate

02 Volume of injectate

03 Size of needle

04 Speed of injection

05 Route and site of injection

Fig. 2. Multiple factors are involved in whether or not an SC or IM injection will evoke an aversive reaction by the patient.

osteosarcoma, have an altered somatosensory system and lowered thresholds to noxious stimuli.[53–55] Many patients scheduled for euthanasia are likely to fall into this category. In these cases, veterinarians should be prepared for a response to injection. In children, topical local anesthetic creams often are used to reduce pain and distress of injections but have the disadvantage of taking time to work (from 20 to 40 minutes). A similar approach has been used in cats for IV catheterization.[56] A vibrating cold device was as effective as 4% topical lidocaine cream for IV catheter placement in children and decreased the time for the procedure from a median of 40.5 minutes to 3 minutes.[57] This strategy, which has also been used for IM injections, has not yet been reported in dogs or cats.

Most clinicians have a preferred site for IM injection, but is there a clinically significant difference in the onset and quality of sedation based on that choice? The influence of muscle group on these 2 variables has been studied. In a randomized crossover study, 7 dogs received the same dose of dexmedetomidine and hydromorphone into the semimembranosus, cervical, gluteal, or lumbar muscle groups and were observed by 16 blinded individuals.[58] The sedation score was highest when the semimembranosus group was used; the time to sedation was fastest at the semimembranosus and cervical sites (median times, 5.50 minutes and 6.37 minutes, respectively) compared with the gluteal and lumbar muscles (8.00 minutes and 6.45 minutes, respectively).[58] The same results may not occur with other drugs or drug combinations, but, based on the report of substantial pain reactions to injection at the quadriceps and triceps muscles,[59] the semimembranosus muscle appears to be a good choice. Another advantage of this location is that compared with other locations it is easier to hide what is being done from owners who are present.

SPECIAL CASES

Dogs and cats that have a seizure disorder benefit from having midazolam in their sedation protocol; this acts as a prophylactic measure. Acepromazine can be used in these patients because it does not lower the seizure threshold, as was previously stated in many textbooks.[60] Midazolam provides excellent muscle relaxations so is a beneficial addition to any pre-euthanasia sedation protocol in cats and dogs.

Patients in heart failure have a lower cardiac output and slower circulation time. After IV administration of a drug, the peak blood concentration is determined by the dose, the rate of administration, and the cardiac output.[61] A low cardiac output results in a higher peak concentration in blood because the drug is mixed with a smaller volume of blood during administration.[61] It takes longer, however, to reach its site of action, the brain. If an anesthetic induction agent is injected with the goal of the animal waking up, a lower dose is given on a milligrams/kilogram basis61, for euthanasia, there is no need to lower the dose of pentobarbital or pentobarbital and phenytoin (discussed later), but extra time must be allowed for the drug to take effect and inform owners that their pet may take longer to pass.

Patients in respiratory distress benefit greatly by being sedated. Acepromazine and opioids (eg, butorphanol) are ideal in this patent population. In humans, opioids frequently are prescribed for breathlessness at the end of life, although their exact mechanism of action is uncertain. A neuroleptic combination of an opioid and acepromazine can relieve the aversive effects of breathlessness and many dyspneic patients become calmer after sedation.

INTRAVENOUS EUTHANASIA

Using only the IV route for euthanasia is still common practice. This requires gaining IV access in a nonsedated dog or cat, which may or may not be easy and many cause pain and distress to the patient. In many instances the pet is separated from the owner to place an IV catheter and this is far from ideal at a time when the human-animal bond is fragile, and owners wish to spend every last precious moment with their pet. Unless an IV catheter is already in place for another reason, this technique is not advised. If the IV route is used, it is still prudent to sedate the animal so that the owner has time to spend with it; a 1-step euthanasia process is very sudden and less acceptable to most owners.

A major drawback of not using presedation and anesthesia protocols is that if gaining IV access is unsuccessful, alternative routes are limited, impractical, and undesirable (eg, intraperitoneal injection [dogs and cats] and intrahepatic injection in cats only). Another disadvantage of omitting the sedation step is that the various stages of anesthesia are more likely to be exhibited during the injection of euthanasia solutions: these include vocalization, excitement, and movement. Failure to gain IV access necessitates administering appropriate drugs that permits the clinician to proceed with euthanasia.

THE EFFECT OF PROPOFOL ADMINISTERED PRIOR TO ADMINISTRATION OF A PENTOBARBITAL-PHENYTOIN SOLUTION

In a prospective study, 446 client-owned dogs were enrolled and randomly assigned to receive propofol prior to a pentobarbital-phenytoin (group PPP; n = 200) or pentobarbital-phenytoin alone (group PP; n = 246) for euthanasia.[62] The study was conducted because of the awareness of undesirable side effects, including but not limited to, agonal breaths, vocalization, and muscle activity during euthanasia, which are distressing to observe, and because of the lack of studies available on how to mitigate these. The protocol used involved placing an IV catheter then administering approximately 5 mg/kg (4.5 mg/kg ± 2.9 [mean ± SD]) of propofol over 5 seconds to 30 seconds, followed by PP, or giving PP alone over 30 seconds to 60 seconds. The dose of pentobarbital and phenytoin was 182.6 mg/kg ± 109.8 (mean ± SD) in the propofol group and 166.9 mg/kg ± 105.6 (mean ± SD) in the PP group; there was no statistical difference in the dose between groups, with both given a wide range. Seven specific adverse events were recoded if they happened and a euthanasia score was calculated based on summation of these events. The percentage of dogs exhibiting 1 or more adverse events was 26.5% in the PPP group and 35.2% on the PP group, with no statistically significant difference in euthanasia scores between the 2 protocols.[62] The only difference between groups was a lower incidence of perimortem muscle activity; with propofol this occurred 6% of the time versus 14% when it was not used.

EUTHANASIA SOLUTIONS

The types of euthanasia solutions that are commercially available along with their pros and cons have recently been discussed elsewhere[1] and are not discussed in this article.

DRUG SHORTAGES

All practitioners should have a backup plan for temporary or permanent unavailability of drugs they use for sedation, anesthesia, and euthanasia. This is an era of drug shortages, which are a result of several factors, including production sites failing inspection and the impact of natural disasters, such as hurricanes. Therefore, veterinarians need to be prepared, be agile, and think outside the box if 1 of the drugs normally used suddenly becomes unavailable. Updates on drug shortages are reported by the Food and Drug Administraiton.[63,64] Ideally clinicians should be familiar with at least 2 sedation and anesthesia protocols for dogs and cats. If euthanasia solutions are unavailable, IV potassium chloride can be used in anesthetized animals.[2] Potassium chloride causes cardiac arrest and recommended doses are 1 mmol/kg to 2 mmol/kg (1–2 mEq/kg), equivalent to 75 mg/kg to 150 mg/kg. Potassium chloride is commercially available, easier to administer, and has a faster onset of action, so is preferred to magnesium sulfate.

An alternative is to use an overdose of an anesthetic agent. Propofol is a practical choice because of its availability and low therapeutic index; the therapeutic index is the lethal or toxic dose divided by the effective dose in 50% of the test population. Compared with alfaxalone and ketamine, propofol has a narrow therapeutic margin; therefore, relatively small volumes are required to produce an anesthetic overdose and death, especially if it is given rapidly.[65–67]

SUMMARY

The act of euthanasia can have far-reaching effects on owners and those who perform it and, in some cases, can be distressing for patients. Providing sedation or anesthesia prior to euthanasia has many benefits. Despite euthanasia being the last appointment for most dogs and cats, veterinarians have a limited evidence base to guide them on the choice of the best sedation or anesthesia protocol prior to euthanasia in a population with a diverse health and behavioral status. In part due to the increased awareness of the benefits of low stress handling of veterinary patients, several drugs that can be given by the oral, OTM, and buccal routes to facilitate transport and clinical examination have been identified and can be included in euthanasia protocols to decrease stress for the patient and increase acceptability for the owners. Veterinarians must continue to look, however, for better ways to perform euthanasia. The veterinary profession has been given the unique honor to legally perform euthanasia to relieve animal suffering and veterinarians owe it to patients and their families to perfect how the final appointment plays out.

DISCLOSURE

Jurox Animal Health is the manufacturer and distributer of alfaxalone (Alfaxan Multidose), which is an anesthetic discussed in the article. The author is a consultant (a member of the Jurox Anesthesia Advisory Board) for this company.

REFERENCES

1. Marchitelli B. An objective exploration of euthanasia and adverse events. Vet Clin North Am Small Anim Pract 2019;49(3):553–63.
2. AVMA guidelines for the Euthanasia of animals: 2020 Edition. Available at: www.avma.org/resources-tools/avma-policies/avma-guidelines-euthanasia-animals. Accessed January 20, 2020.
3. Tranquilli WJ, Grimm KA. Introduction: use, definitions, history, concepts, classification, and considerations for anesthesia and analgesia. In: Grimm KA, Lamont LA, Tranquilli WJ, et al, editors. Veterinary anesthesia and analagesia. The fifth edition of lumb and jones. 5th edition. Ames (IA): John Wiley & Sons, Inc; 2015. p. 3–10.
4. Siao KT, Pypendop BH, Ilkiw JE. Pharmacokinetics of gabapentin in cats. Am J Vet Res 2010;71(7):817–21.
5. Adrian D, Papich MG, Baynes R, et al. The pharmacokinetics of gabapentin in cats. J Vet Intern Med 2018;32(6):1996–2002.
6. van Haaften KA, Forsythe LRE, Stelow EA, et al. Effects of a single preappointment dose of gabapentin on signs of stress in cats during transportation and veterinary examination. J Am Vet Med Assoc 2017;251(10):1175–81.
7. Pankratz KE, Ferris KK, Griffith EH, et al. Use of single-dose oral gabapentin to attenuate fear responses in cage-trap confined community cats: a double-blind, placebo-controlled field trial. J Feline Med Surg 2018;20(6):535–43.
8. Impellizzeri P, Vinci E, Gugliandolo MC, et al. Premedication with melatonin vs midazolam: efficacy on anxiety and compliance in paediatric surgical patients. Eur J Pediatr 2017;176(7):947–53.
9. Niggemann JR, Tichy A, Eberspacher-Schweda MC, et al. Preoperative calming effect of melatonin and its influence on propofol dose for anesthesia induction in healthy dogs. Vet Anaesth Analg 2019;46(5):560–7.
10. Chill protocol to manage aggressive & fearful dogs. Available at: www.cliniciansbrief.com/article/chill-protocol-manage-aggressive-fearful-dogs. Accessed November 12, 2019.
11. Orlando JM, Case BC, Thomson AE, et al. Use of oral trazodone for sedation in cats: a pilot study. J Feline Med Surg 2016;18(6):476–82.
12. Stevens BJ, Frantz EM, Orlando JM, et al. Efficacy of a single dose of trazodone hydrochloride given to cats prior to veterinary visits to reduce signs of transport- and examination-related anxiety. J Am Vet Med Assoc 2016;249(2):202–7.
13. Gilbert-Gregory SE, Stull JW, Rice MR, et al. Effects of trazodone on behavioral signs of stress in hospitalized dogs. J Am Vet Med Assoc 2016;249(11):1281–91.
14. Jay AR, Krotscheck U, Parsley E, et al. Pharmacokinetics, bioavailability, and hemodynamic effects of trazodone after intravenous and oral administration of a single dose to dogs. Am J Vet Res 2013;74(11):1450–6.
15. Gruen ME, Roe SC, Griffith E, et al. Use of trazodone to facilitate postsurgical confinement in dogs. J Am Vet Med Assoc 2014;245(3):296–301.
16. Ramsay EC, Wetzel RW. Comparison of five regimens for oral administration of medication to induce sedation in dogs prior to euthanasia. J Am Vet Med Assoc 1998;213(2):240–2.
17. Smith AJ. Tips and gentle tricks providing euthanasia under challenging circumstances; IAAHPC proceedings notes 2018. Available at: https://learn.iaahpc.org. Accessed October 18, 2019.

18. Huang HC, Huang SW, Yu KH, et al. Development of a sedation protocol using orally administered tiletamine-zolazepam-acepromazine in free-roaming dogs. Vet Anaesth Analg 2017;44(5):1035–41.
19. Hashem A, Kietzmann M, Scherkl R. The pharmacokinetics and bioavailability of acepromazine in the plasma of dogs. Dtsch Tierarztl Wochenschr 1992;99(10): 396–8 [in German].
20. Robertson SA, Taylor PM, Sear JW. Systemic uptake of buprenorphine by cats after oral mucosal administration. Vet Rec 2003;152(22):675–8.
21. Robertson SA, Lascelles BD, Taylor PM, et al. PK-PD modeling of buprenorphine in cats: intravenous and oral transmucosal administration. J Vet Pharmacol Ther 2005;28(5):453–60.
22. Giordano T, Steagall PV, Ferreira TH, et al. Postoperative analgesic effects of intravenous, intramuscular, subcutaneous or oral transmucosal buprenorphine administered to cats undergoing ovariohysterectomy. Vet Anaesth Analg 2010; 37(4):357–66.
23. Bortolami E, Slingsby L, Love EJ. Comparison of two formulations of buprenorphine in cats administered by the oral transmucosal route. J Feline Med Surg 2012;14(8):534–9.
24. Abbo LA, Ko JC, Maxwell LK, et al. Pharmacokinetics of buprenorphine following intravenous and oral transmucosal administration in dogs. Vet Ther 2008;9(2): 83–93.
25. Slingsby LS, Taylor PM, Monroe T. Thermal antinociception after dexmedetomidine administration in cats: a comparison between intramuscular and oral transmucosal administration. J Feline Med Surg 2009;11(10):829–34.
26. Porters N, Bosmans T, Debille M, et al. Sedative and antinociceptive effects of dexmedetomidine and buprenorphine after oral transmucosal or intramuscular administration in cats. Vet Anaesth Analg 2014;41(1):90–6.
27. Cohen AE, Bennett SL. Oral transmucosal administration of dexmedetomidine for sedation in 4 dogs. Can Vet J 2015;56(11):1144–8.
28. Dent BT, Aarnes TK, Wavreille VA, et al. Pharmacokinetics and pharmacodynamic effects of oral transmucosal and intravenous administration of dexmedetomidine in dogs. Am J Vet Res 2019;80(10):969–75.
29. Messenger KM, Hopfensperger M, Knych HK, et al. Pharmacokinetics of detomidine following intravenous or oral-transmucosal administration and sedative effects of the oral-transmucosal treatment in dogs. Am J Vet Res 2016;77(4): 413–20.
30. Hopfensperger M, Messenger KM, Papich MG, et al. The use of oral transmucosal detomidine hydrochloride gel to facilitate handling in dogs. J Vet Behav 2013;8(3):114–23.
31. Available at: www.merckvetmanual.com/special-subjects/reference-guides/weight-to-body-surface-area-conversion-for-dogs. Accessed August 12, 2019.
32. Wetzel RW, Ramsay EC. Comparison of four regimens for intraoral administration of medication to induce sedation in cats prior to euthanasia. J Am Vet Med Assoc 1998;213(2):243–5.
33. Nejamkin P, Cavilla V, Clausse M, et al. Sedative and physiologic effects of tiletamine-zolazepam following buccal administration in cats. J Feline Med Surg 2019. https://doi.org/10.1177/1098612x19827116.
34. Micieli F, Santangelo B, Reynaud F, et al. Sedative and cardiovascular effects of intranasal or intramuscular dexmedetomidine in healthy dogs. Vet Anaesth Analg 2017;44(4):703–9.

35. Jafarbeglou M, Marjani M. Comparison of the sedative effects of medetomidine administered intranasally, by atomization or drops, and intramuscular injection in dogs. Vet Anaesth Analg 2019;46(6):815–9.
36. Santos LC, Ludders JW, Erb HN, et al. A randomized, blinded, controlled trial of the antiemetic effect of ondansetron on dexmedetomidine-induced emesis in cats. Vet Anaesth Analg 2011;38(4):320–7.
37. Ko JC, Berman AG. Anesthesia in shelter medicine. Top Companion Anim Med 2010;25(2):92–7.
38. Ko JC, Austin BR, Barletta M, et al. Evaluation of dexmedetomidine and ketamine in combination with various opioids as injectable anesthetic combinations for castration in cats. J Am Vet Med Assoc 2011;239(11):1453–62.
39. Polson S, Taylor PM, Yates D. Analgesia after feline ovariohysterectomy under midazolam-medetomidine-ketamine anaesthesia with buprenorphine or butorphanol, and carprofen or meloxicam: a prospective, randomised clinical trial. J Feline Med Surg 2012;14(8):553–9.
40. Williams LS, Levy JK, Robertson SA, et al. Use of the anesthetic combination of tiletamine, zolazepam, ketamine, and xylazine for neutering feral cats. J Am Vet Med Assoc 2002;220(10):1491–5.
41. Lap of Love resources password DVMSUPPORT. Available at: www.lapoflove.com/resources. Accessed November 20, 2019.
42. Alfaxalone safety data sheet pH ~ 7. Available at: www.jurox.com/us/product/alfaxan. Accessed August 15, 2019.
43. Khenissi L, Nikolayenkova-Topie O, Broussaud S, et al. Comparison of intramuscular alfaxalone and ketamine combined with dexmedetomidine and butorphanol for castration in cats. J Feline Med Surg 2017;19(8):791–7.
44. Granfone MC, Walker JM, Smith LJ. Evaluation of an intramuscular butorphanol and alfaxalone protocol for feline blood donation: a pilot study. J Feline Med Surg 2018;20(8):793–8.
45. Reader RC, Barton BA, Abelson AL. Comparison of two intramuscular sedation protocols on sedation, recovery and ease of venipuncture for cats undergoing blood donation. J Feline Med Surg 2019;21(2):95–102.
46. Ribas T, Bublot I, Junot S, et al. Effects of intramuscular sedation with alfaxalone and butorphanol on echocardiographic measurements in healthy cats. J Feline Med Surg 2015;17(6):530–6.
47. Deutsch J, Jolliffe C, Archer E, et al. Intramuscular injection of alfaxalone in combination with butorphanol for sedation in cats. Vet Anaesth Analg 2017;44(4):794–802.
48. Patterson M, Caulkett N, neuhaus P, et al. A Novel Formulation of Alfaxalaone Increases the Utility for Remote Delivery in Bighorn Sheep (Ovis canadensis). Paper presented at: Joint EAZWV/AAZV/Leibniz-IZW Conference. Prague, Czech Republic, October 6, 2018.
49. Ramoo S, Bradbury LA, Anderson GA, et al. Sedation of hyperthyroid cats with subcutaneous administration of a combination of alfaxalone and butorphanol. Aust Vet J 2013;91(4):131–6.
50. Tamura J, Ishizuka T, Fukui S, et al. The pharmacological effects of the anesthetic alfaxalone after intramuscular administration to dogs. J Vet Med Sci 2015;77(3):289–96.
51. Maney JK. Sedative and physiologic effects of low-dose intramuscular alfaxalone in dogs. Vet Anaesth Analg 2017;44(5):1184–8.

52. Cruz-Benedetti IC, Bublot I, Ribas T, et al. Pharmacokinetics of intramuscular al-faxalone and its echocardiographic, cardiopulmonary and sedative effects in healthy dogs. PLoS One 2018;13(9):e0204553.
53. Guillot M, Taylor PM, Rialland P, et al. Evoked temporal summation in cats to high-light central sensitization related to osteoarthritis-associated chronic pain: a pre-liminary study. PLoS One 2014;9(5):e97347.
54. Knazovicky D, Helgeson ES, Case B, et al. Widespread somatosensory sensitivity in naturally occurring canine model of osteoarthritis. Pain 2016;157(6):1325–32.
55. Monteiro BP, de Lorimier LP, Moreau M, et al. Pain characterization and response to palliative care in dogs with naturally-occurring appendicular osteosarcoma: an open label clinical trial. PLoS One 2018;13(12):e0207200.
56. Oliveira RL, Soares JH, Moreira CM, et al. The effects of lidocaine-prilocaine cream on responses to intravenous catheter placement in cats sedated with dex-medetomidine and either methadone or nalbuphine. Vet Anaesth Analg 2019; 46(4):492–5.
57. Potts DA, Davis KF, Elci OU, et al. A vibrating cold device to reduce pain in the pediatric emergency department: a randomized clinical trial. Pediatr Emerg Care 2019;35(6):419–25.
58. Carter JE, Lewis C, Beths T. Onset and quality of sedation after intramuscular administration of dexmedetomidine and hydromorphone in various muscle groups in dogs. J Am Vet Med Assoc 2013;243(11):1569–72.
59. Self IA, Hughes JM, Kenny DA, et al. Effect of muscle injection site on preanaes-thetic sedation in dogs. Vet Rec 2009;164(11):323–6.
60. Tobias KM, Marioni-Henry K, Wagner R. A retrospective study on the use of ace-promazine maleate in dogs with seizures. J Am Anim Hosp Assoc 2006;42(4): 283–9.
61. Roberts F, Freshwater-Turner D. Pharmacokinetics and anaesthesia. Cont Educ Anaesth Crit Care Pain 2007;7(1):25–9.
62. Bullock JM, Lanaux TM, Shmalberg JW. Comparison of pentobarbital-phenytoin alone vs propofol prior to pentobarbital-phenytoin for euthanasia in 436 client-owned dogs. J Vet Emerg Crit Care (San Antonio) 2019;29(2):161–5.
63. Drug shortages. Available at: www.accessdata.fda.gov/scripts/drugshortages/dsp_SearchResults.cfm. Accessed December 22, 2019.
64. Muir W, Lerche P, Wiese A, et al. Cardiorespiratory and anesthetic effects of clin-ical and supraclinical doses of alfaxalone in dogs. Vet Anaesth Analg 2008;35(6): 451–62.
65. Muir W, Lerche P, Wiese A, et al. The cardiorespiratory and anesthetic effects of clinical and supraclinical doses of alfaxalone in cats. Vet Anaesth Analg 2009; 36(1):42–54.
66. Zanos P, Moaddel R, Morris PJ, et al. Ketamine and ketamine metabolite pharma-cology: insights into therapeutic mechanisms. Pharmacol Rev 2018;70(3): 621–60.
67. Sahinovic MM, Struys M, Absalom AR. Clinical pharmacokinetics and pharmaco-dynamics of propofol. Clin Pharmacokinet 2018;57(12):1539–58.

Common and Alternative Routes of Euthanasia Solution Administration

Kathleen Cooney, DVM, MS, CHPV, CCFP

KEYWORDS

- Euthanasia • Barbiturates • Euthanasia agents • Intravenous • Intracardiac
- Intrahepatic • Intrarenal • Intraperitoneal

KEY POINTS

- There are many acceptable routes of euthanasia solution administration for companion animals.
- The best method is the one that matches the patient's signalment, practitioner skill, and available supplies, with consideration of all known criteria.
- Alternative methods are available and will continue to evolve with animal welfare and research.

INTRODUCTION

The administration of a solution to elicit death remains the gold standard in companion animal euthanasia. Depending on the type of solution, death is achieved via either direct depression of neurons (necessary for life) in the central nervous system or through hypoxia. In this article, we explore the most common drugs used in small animal practice and the manner in which euthanasia is accomplished. We review the current preferred techniques as well as some up and coming alternatives in modern practice. What remains most important is the gentle acceptance of death by the patient and the ability of loved ones to be nearby for support (**Box 1**).

EUTHANASIA SOLUTIONS OF TODAY

In small animal clinical work, there is a limited number of euthanasia drugs available for use, in particular owing to the need to both facilitate a gentle, efficient death event and ensure those present witness minimal side effects. All anesthetic drugs have an overdose threshold, but only a few are well-suited to everyday euthanasia,

Companion Animal Euthanasia Training Academy, 8466 Golden Fields Lane, Loveland, CO 80538, USA
E-mail address: cooneydvm@gmail.com

Vet Clin Small Anim 50 (2020) 545–560
https://doi.org/10.1016/j.cvsm.2019.12.005

Box 1	
Common routes of solution administration	
Intravenous	IV
Intracardiac	IC
Intrahepatic	IH
Intrarenal	IR
Intraperitoneal	IP
Oral	PO

namely, the barbiturates. As discussed in Kathleen Cooney's article, "Historical Perspective of Euthanasia in Veterinary Medicine," in this issue, barbiturates remain the standard drug type to reach for. It is worth noting that, as of 2020, pure barbiturates are not approved by the US Food and Drug Administration owing to their Schedule II classification; however, drugs like Vortech Pharmaceutical's Fatal Plus are listed in compliance with manufacturing requirements.[1] Schedule III barbiturates (those with additives) are FDA approved, but are only approved for canines, even though it is commonplace to use them off-label for all species. Barbiturates readily available (at present) have the potential for expedient cardiac death, are reasonably priced, and produce minimal signs of active death that may be hard for owners to watch. Although other drugs can be equally as available, most have other factors that reduce their standings in the lineup, including their lack of formal approval as euthanasia agents. Examples include the overdosing of dissociatives (ketamine), neurosteroids (alfaxalone), benzodiazepines (midazolam), and opioids (carfentanil citrate). The American Veterinary Medical Association has gone to great length to assist practitioners in knowing which drugs are acceptable, acceptable with conditions, and unacceptable. For our purposes here, we focus only on those drugs used in everyday practice and times when nontraditional drugs are necessary.

There are a few substances that may be needed as alternatives to traditional anesthetic drugs used for euthanasia purposes, namely, magnesium sulfate and potassium chloride. These drugs are considered compounded when used for euthanasia purposes, such as being added to water to saturation points before administration and are not approved by the FDA as euthanasia agents. They are worth knowing about, but not advocated for in traditional practice under normal circumstances. Doses for barbiturates are shared in the Routes of Administration sections, and other drugs are listed here.

1. Barbiturates: These agents are widely recognized as best practice because they are rapid acting, can be administered through various routes, and have a high percentage of reliability and irreversibility when given properly.[2] Barbiturates work on the central nervous system as gamma aminobutyric acid potentiators. They are considered super potent anesthetics, acting on various inhibitory pathways so effectively that the time to death (TTD) is expected in less than 1 minute when properly dosed directly into the venous system. Barbiturates are very short acting, meaning an animal will revive in 4 to 6 hours if not properly advanced through all stages of anesthesia. Pure barbiturates are those containing pentobarbital with no additives and are class II controlled drugs. Typical concentrations range from 200 to 390 mg/mL. In the US, 390mg/ml is the standard product concentration, and all doses listed in this chapter on based on it. Desirable barbiturates are those that are potent, nonirritating, stable in solution, and inexpensive. Sodium pentobarbital best fits these criteria and is most widely used, although others such as secobarbital are also acceptable.[3] Their biggest pitfall remains the contamination of the

body following death. Barbiturate-laden carcasses remain a tangible threat when ingested by other living animals or when there is concern of soil contamination.

2. Barbiturate-combination products: This group includes those with additives, such as phenytoin sodium or lidocaine, and are typically class III controlled drugs. The additive is designed to reduce the controlled nature of the euthanasia solution making it easier to obtain and store. The additive, usually with human-injury properties like being cardiotoxic, reduces the likelihood it would be abused as a sleep aid or a method of getting high. Depending on the type of additive, the routes of administration may be affected. Lidocaine has shown numbing and absorption benefits, and is likely to become a more common additive than is currently available today.[4] Phenytoin sodium can be used by itself to facilitate death, but only in unconscious patients (common in countries with no access to barbiturates.

3. Overdosing nonbarbiturate anesthetics: Anesthetics that work on the central nervous system and are used for surgical induction will all have a lethal dose. However, the exact volume and rate of administration to achieve death remains largely unstudied and is likely not a viable option in most situations. Overdosing nonbarbiturate anesthetics would be considered desperate and undesirable because they are not FDA approved for euthanasia nor well-understood. Examples include ketamine, tiletamine, propofol, and alfaxalone. An animal would be rendered unconscious with smaller doses, then pushed to the point of overdose. They are generally considered unnecessary to use in most animals owing to the availability of barbiturates and potentially less expensive alternatives. Other examples of drugs one might consider with no other options include α2-agonists, benzodiazepines, or opioids but limited study has been conducted on the efficacy of their use and is generally not recommended when other, more predictable agents are available. Lidocaine is an anesthetic being discussed more of late, particularly in horses.[5] It is possible there is application in small animals, but further study is needed.

4. Potassium chloride and magnesium sulfate (not common in small animals). Potassium chloride (KCl) is a hypoxia agent rather than an anesthetic. It works to stop the heart directly and therefore requires the animal be in a state of complete unconsciousness beforehand; unaware the heart is ceasing to beat which would cause extreme pain and anxiety. It may only be given intravenous (IV) or intracardiac (IC). A saturated solution of KCl can be prepared by mixing 350 to 560 g of KCl in 1 liter of warm water and stirring. KCl is an adjunctive method in many species and only used when barbiturates are unavailable or when a body cannot be safely disposed of. Typically dosing is 1 to 2 mmol/kg, 75 to 150 mg/kg, or 1 to 2 mEq K^+/ kg. KCl often leads to active signs of dying such as agonal breathing, opisthotonos stretching, and twitching. Magnesium sulfate ($MgSO_4$) also leads to death when the preferred barbiturates are not available or practical. It must be given IV with the animal unconscious similar to KCl. The solution is made my combining approximately 350 g or enough to saturate a liter of water at room temperature. The dose is to effect, meaning it is administered until the heart stops. Death is typical in less than 5 minutes. Because $MgSO_4$ has fewer active signs of dying compared with KCl, it could be considered the preferable choice between the two. Note that there are limited studies on $MgSO_4$ use in small animals, with most dating back to the last century.

CHOOSING THE RIGHT METHOD

The method of euthanasia to choose for a patient depends on many factors. Most important are the following considerations, including the patient's comfort with minimalization of pain and distress. As we will see when reading on, intraorgan injections are increasing in popularity. High perfusion of the tissue and ease of isolation and administration make them useful in many situations.

1. Comfort with the technique: It is advisable to select a method that one is familiar with, especially when clients and loved ones are gathered close, keeping in mind that the best method may be one requiring a profession to step outside their comfort zone.
2. Presence of pre-euthanasia sedation or anesthesia: There are certain administration techniques that may only be carried out with the patient in a state of unconsciousness.
3. Supplies on hand: Some methods of administration require unique medical supplies to be successful. Plenty of everything is best readied before the appointment even begins.
4. Type of euthanasia solution you use and amount you have available: Not all types of solutions/drugs are appropriate for every method. The volume of solution needs adjustment depending on the method.
5. Signalment and physical condition of the patient: A patient's emotional and physical health should be considered in method selection. Here are some illustrations to the point.
   a. Weight: Overweight patients are not well-suited to intraperitoneal (IP) injections.
   b. Size: The larger the patient, the more solution must be available.
   c. Age: Older patients may lead to advanced states of poor health and subsequent difficulties with injections.
   d. Disease: Disease may affect how quickly solution is circulated around the body to its target location.
   e. Species: Some species must be euthanized in unique ways, or adjunctive methods embraced to facilitate death, for example, reptiles.
   f. Breeds: Short legged dogs have less vein to work with than their taller counterparts.
6. The need for a postmortem examination: If there is need to examine the body after euthanasia, specifically to look at 1 organ or another, the method selected should avoid the organ altogether.

THE GROWING TREND OF INTRAORGAN INJECTIONS

There is a change brewing in the world of companion animal euthanasia. More and more veterinarians and technicians are shifting toward intraorgan injections as their preferred method over IV administration, especially those who specialize in end-of-life–related veterinary work. An opinion poll taken at the 2018 International Association for Animal Hospice and Palliative Care conference in Tempe, Arizona, revealed some perspective. Eighty-three veterinarians participated in a survey asking about their preferred method of euthanasia for dogs and cats, and why they preferred one technique over another. Although the group of respondents was small, they represented varied backgrounds in mobile and hospital settings and are largely focused on improving the euthanasia experience for their clients and patients.

Of the 83 respondents, the favorite euthanasia technique for dogs remained IV injections. Ranked second was intrahepatic (IH), but when chosen, this one was considered most effective in smaller dogs. Very few ranked it as preferred in larger dogs. Coming in third was IC, of which a few practitioners claimed it as their preferred technique even over IV. Intrarenal (IR) and IP injections were also chosen, but they regularly came in last place. In cats, the preferred technique was also IV injections, but a close

---

Box 2
Intraorgan injections

Opinions behind intraorgan injection preference
1. No time concerns
2. Clients *seem to be* comfortable with it
3. The practitioner likes more options
4. Intraorgan injections are simple; no need to search for a vein

Opinions on why to avoid intraorgan injections
1. Lack of training or familiarity, especially in the presence of clients
2. Distrust over efficiency and shorter TTD (risk of longer appointment time)
3. Desire to avoid pre-euthanasia sedation/anesthesia

---

second was the IR injection. Many indicated IR injections were their preferred route in all cats, except those who were overweight or in times when the kidneys could not be isolated. IH injections for cats came in third and IC and IP injections were last. So although many still preferred IV injections, many claimed to have switched over to intraorgan injections and only rarely reach for a vein (**Box 2**).[6]

Although most in this small study said they still preferred IV injections, 34% say they prefer intraorgan injections whenever possible. If intraorgan routes are to continue in acceptance, there needs to be increased euthanasia technique training, better euthanasia education as a whole leading to improved confidence by the practitioner, and longer preplanned appointment times.

COMMON ROUTES OF ADMINISTRATION
Intravenous Injection

An IV injection means the solution is being delivered directly into a vein. Which vein to work with depends in part on the veterinary team's preference and the patient's physical characteristics. To perform an IV euthanasia, the veterinarian or staff member will need to find a vein and either place an indwelling catheter, use a butterfly catheter, or attempt direct venipuncture. The most common veins to use include the cephalic, medial (cats) and lateral (dogs) saphenous, and dorsal pedal vein. Other available but less sought after veins include the jugular, ventral abdominal, or ear vein, depending on the species of interest. Each has its pros and cons. The administrator should pick the one that is most appropriate under the circumstances (**Fig. 1**).

Limb veins are superficial just under the skin and often visible. It is advised to shave fur from the area to increase this visibility and make injections more straightforward. Shaving also helps the team to understand a patient's depth of sleep before attempting to insert a needle, such as when the patient has already been given a sedative beforehand. A vein can be easy to isolate or they may be difficult to control, meaning it may take multiple attempts before the team is convinced the vein is useable. If the first vein of choice is not suitable, another vein can be tried. This author recommends trying no more than a few times to find a vein before moving on to an intraorgan injection.

The placement of an indwelling catheter in the vein is considered the safest approach regardless if the patient is asleep or awake. Catheters help to ensure that the euthanasia solution given will not accidently be placed outside of the vein, as can happen with direct venipuncture. Needles or butterfly catheters create a risk of the needle puncturing through the vein at any time. Catheter placement opens up the option to offer the client more privacy before proceeding with the euthanasia, without further concerns of dropping blood pressures (**Box 3**).

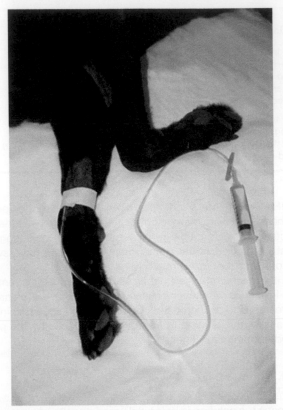

Fig. 1. IV catheter placement in a dog with extension set. (*Courtesy of* Kathleen Cooney, DVM Loveland, Colorado.)

The standard barbiturate injection amount is 1 mL per 10 lb (4.5 kg) body weight for all mammals and birds.[2] Reptiles may require more. If the exact weight of the patient is unknown, one must make the best educated guess. It is advisable to give at least 2 mL more than the required amount, especially if the exact weight is unknown.[5] Giving

---

Box 3
Tips for improved IV administration

Use most visible and palpable vein

Clip/shave fur

Have all supplies available and ready to use

Choose Luer-locking syringes

Use a good tourniquet or skilled assistant

Squeeze the limb to increase blood volume at site

Avoid rubbing alcohol to aid in visualizing the vein (aversive smell)

Test for proper placement before administering euthanasia solution

Only try 1 or 2 times before moving to another method (decreases waiting time for the client)

more than recommended is acceptable for any kind of euthanasia solution given. When performing an IV injection, death occurs very quickly. The onset of death with a barbiturate should be seen within 30 seconds or so.[7]

Technical challenges may arise with IV administration, such as when the veins are difficult to isolate owing to poor blood pressure or the skin is thick and/or loose in the area. It can take great patience to work with a challenging vein and whenever practical, the most skilled phlebotomist on site should be brought in. Another tricky scenario is extravasation of the solution outside of the vein. If a bleb is seen forming in the surrounding tissue, the needle or catheter has slipped out of the vein. The team will have to decide if it is best to try again somewhere else along the vein or move on to another method.

Intracardiac Injection

The administration of barbiturates, or any anesthetic affecting the brain, is most efficient when delivered into the heart. The heart is in closest proximity to the head compared with the rest of the common injection sites. In fact, with respect to euthanasia, the heart is used as nothing more than a large vessel to move the anesthetics along to the brain. TTD is rapid and the dosing of barbiturates is 1 mL per 10 lb (4.5 kg), the same as IV. Although IC injections are indeed very efficient, they remain less chosen compared with IV owing to the ease of missing the injection site, the need to draw back blood to check for proper placement, and the sentimental nature of the heart itself.

IC injections have been used in small animal euthanasia from the very beginning of veterinary medicine. It is well-known today that IC injections on awake animals cause pain and, therefore, all patients must be unconscious before proceeding with insertion of the needle; however, in the first half of the 20th century, it was common to inject the heart in conscious patients.[8] An unconscious state prevents the patient from feeling anything, including the common need to move the needle around and redirect until blood is located.

The goal is to locate the heart using landmarks such as the point of maximum intensity, where the heart sounds are readily detectable with stethoscope. The heart beat can also usually be felt by laying one's hands over the region. A needle long enough to reach inside of the heart is required and, depending on the size of the patient, will range from 1 to 4 inches in length. Anywhere in a heart chamber, like the ventricles or atrium, is acceptable to inject. Another landmark is where the olecranon of the elbow would reside near the chest wall if the patient were standing (**Figs. 2 and 3**).

Because the heart is shielded by the rib cage, veterinary teams must know their anatomy and where best to insert the needle. The heart in most dogs and cats will reside from the second or third intercostal space to the fifth or sixth intercostal space, and from the sternum to about two-thirds of the way up the thorax.[9] In this author's experience, the heart is usually more cranial and ventral than one might think. The needle can be attached directly to a syringe with solution or attached to an extension set used to bring the syringe itself away from the body wall.[10] This is advantageous when trying to conceal blood from the client's site. Needle insertion is directed between the ribs.

A unique feature of IC injections compared with others is the need for extra room in the syringe to draw back blood to test for proper placement. There needs to be at least 1 to 2 mL of unused space in the syringe to capture blood from the heart. When the needle is inserted, negative pressure is applied to the syringe to pull in blood. If the heart is missed on the first try, it is possible the suction will pull in air from the lungs

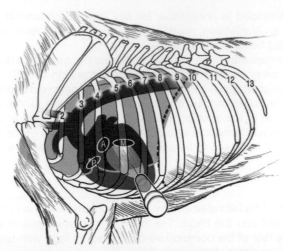

Fig. 2. Left-sided IC injection landmarks in canine patients. A, aortic valve; M, mitral valve; P, pulmonary valve. (*Courtesy of* the CAETA program, Loveland CO.)

or even free fluid in the chest cavity. Extra space in the syringe is a necessity. When blood is found, it will be a rapid intake gush rather than a trickle (**Box 4**).

Technical challenges can occur with this technique, as with any other technique. It is not always easy to locate the heart and multiple attempts may be necessary. Pathology in the thoracic region can change the heart's location, lead to pulmonary effusion, and even change the heart's anatomy, making injection problematic. When the heart cannot be located or the injection does not lead to death in short course, another method can be quickly turned to. Should clients be concerned about the heart being injected, it is appropriate to gently inform them the heart is not being harmed. The heart is simply moving the drug along in the body to the brain. This would not be the case with KCl, which does work to stop the heart directly.

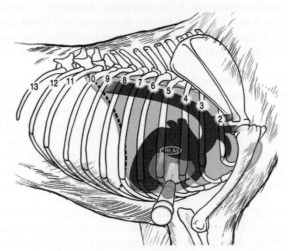

Fig. 3. Right-sided IC injection landmarks in canine patients. Rt. AV, right atrioventricular valve. (*Courtesy of* the CAETA program, Loveland CO.)

> **Box 4**
> **Tips for improved IC administration**
>
> Use a long enough needle to reach the heart
>
> Choose a large-bore needle to allow for ample blood flowback
>
> Draw back blood again mid injection to ensure continued proper placement
>
> Ensure your syringe has enough room for the solution and blood to assess proper placement
>
> Consider use of a small 1-ml extension set hidden in your hand to reduce the client's view
>
> Apply slow and steady negative pressure while the needle is redirected to find blood
>
> If the heart is not located on the first try, obtain more solution and try again

Intrahepatic Injection

IH injections are delivered into the liver. At this time, only barbiturates or barbiturate combination products are suitable for this injection method. Other agents are best delivered IV or IC. The liver is highly vascular and readily moves barbiturates into the bloodstream, shortening TTD compared with IP injections. Because an organ is being injected, patient unconsciousness is required beforehand. The liver is generally a large organ with a large surface area and injectable space.

With the patient in lateral recumbency, the injection landmark is on either side of the xyphoid process. In birds, the breast bone extends quite caudal over the liver making injection more difficult, but not impossible. A needle long enough to reach the liver should be used. With small pets, a 1-inch needle should be adequate, but in larger pets, a 1.5- to 2.0-inch needle may be necessary. The needle should be angled near 45° cranially. The one administering the injection can draw back on the syringe to check for fluid before injecting, but absence of blood does not indicate improper placement. It is most common to simply insert the needle in the proper place at the proper angle and inject (**Figs. 4** and **5**).

The recommended barbiturate dose is 2 mL per 10 lb (4.5 kg).[3] Death should occur within about 2 minutes or so with a well-performed IH injection.[4] The typical injection rate is 1 mL per second or slower. If around the 2-minute mark there is no change in breathing pattern, more solution may be delivered to the same place or slightly

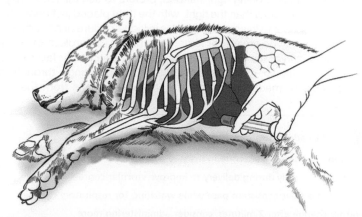

Fig. 4. IH illustration in the canine. (*Courtesy of* the CAETA program, Loveland CO.)

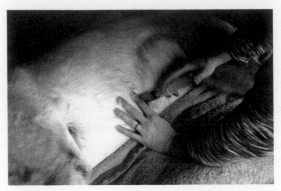

Fig. 5. Demonstration of an IH injection. (*Courtesy of* the CAETA program, Loveland CO.)

adjacent. The needle may be redirected often during delivery of solution to help insure contact with vascular tissue (**Box 5**).

Technical challenges arrive when cessation of breathing and TTD takes longer than expected; 10 minutes or more. It is possible in these cases the liver was missed and an IP injection was completed or the drug was third-spaced somewhere. The spleen is to be avoided because it has been shown to engorge and slow absorption time. It is important to note the liver can be surrounded my adipose tissue and free fluid and, in these circumstances, another method should be reached for first. Many practitioners only reach for IH injections on patients smaller than 50 lbs, although those who are very skilled use it for patients of all sizes.

Intrarenal Injections

IR injections refer to use of the kidneys to uptake the drug into the vascular system. The kidneys, situated in the abdomen, are a viable option for cats and small mammals. In patients with a normal to thin body condition scoring, the kidneys are easy to palpate and isolate for solution administration. When performed correctly, the TTD is usually less than 1 minute, with death common before the injection is even complete. It is an elegant technique allowing the veterinarian to feel the target in their hand. Being a paired organ, it is especially nice when there are two to choose from.

When choosing which kidney to inject, the administrator can use the one they feel and isolate the best. This author, being right-handed, prefers to use the left kidney. In cats, the left kidney sits more caudal than the right, with the right placed just under the last rib. Either kidney is appropriate to inject. If a patient is in kidney failure or has advanced renal disease, the kidneys may be smaller or larger than usual. Regardless of disease, they may be used. The health of the kidney does not dictate success or failure (**Fig. 6**).

To inject, the practitioner inserts the needle with the syringe through the renal capsule into cortical or medullary tissue. A good approach is from the dorsum of

---

Box 5
Tips for improved IH administration

Use a needle long enough to penetrate liver tissue

Redirect the needle slightly during delivery to improve vascular contact

Deliver the drug at a slow, consistent pace while watching for respiratory change

If no respiratory change after 2 minutes, consider administering more

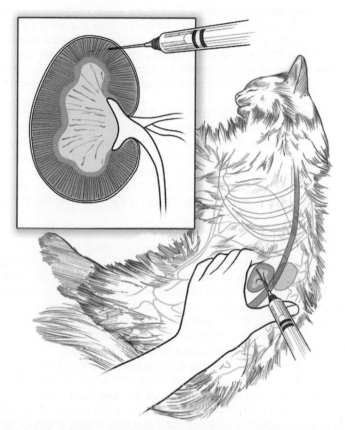

Fig. 6. Illustration showing proper placement of the needle for IR administration. (*Courtesy of* the CAETA program, Loveland CO.)

the patient. A 1-inch needle length of any gauge (larger bore needles are preferred for this and all intraorgan techniques) should be sufficient to easily penetrate the kidney in patients weighing less than 20 lbs in normal body condition. Diseased kidneys can feel granular, cystic, and so on, making needle insertion more difficult. It is best to avoid the renal pelvis because this site may move the euthanasia solution into the ureter and bladder, limiting absorption (**Box 6**).[11]

There is limited knowledge regarding the minimal effect barbiturate dosing for IR injections. The American Veterinary Medical Association Euthanasia Guidelines suggest 3 mL per 10 lb (4.5 kg) with some private practitioners reporting success at 1 mL per 10 lb.[3] This author administers 6 mL per cat with excellent results. Whatever the volume,

Box 6
Tips for improved IR administration
Only attempt injection on a kidney that can be held in place
Feel for swelling, redirect if not properly placed
Inject from the patient's dorsum
If no respiratory change after 1 minute, consider administering more

the kidney should swell owing to increased pressure within the renal capsule. This is the main indication the drug was properly delivered into the renal tissue. Kidney swelling does not guarantee immediate death, but it does increase the odds that death will occur faster.[12] The TTD is very short, at less than 1 minute with this technique. Depending on the volume of solution given, the patient may pass before the injection is complete, adding more merit to less solution being needed than the recommended 3 mL per 10 lbs.

The prevailing challenge with IR injections is accidental release of the kidney mid injection. To prevent this, the administrator needs to have a stabilizing hold and maintain it throughout the entire discharge of solution. If the kidney should slip away, it is acceptable to administer what is left in the syringe into the same area, then acquire more solution and try again. If, on the second attempt, the kidney cannot be found, another organ may be used. Based on a retrospective study in 2011 on IR injections in cats, a second injection within an area of high perfusion should lead to cardiac death within 2 minutes.[12]

Intraperitoneal Injections

IP injections are unique compared with the others described thus far in that they are not directly associated with highly vascular (IV and IC) or well-perfused tissues (IH and IR). Instead the absorption of euthanasia solution is passive across serosal membranes within the abdomen. The speed of solution uptake is greatly dependent on factors like abdominal fluid, hydration status, pathology in the region, and proper placement of the injection itself. IP injections are chosen when other techniques are not possible and when TTD does not have to be as rapid. This method can facilitate death ranging from 5 minutes after injection to more than 1 hour.

To be considered a true IP injection, the solution must be placed in free space within the abdomen. All neighboring organs, including the stomach, intestines, liver, and kidneys, must be avoided, especially in conscious animals. Barbiturates are the only euthanasia agents approved for IP injections, and in particular pure sodium pentobarbital without phenytoin sodium. The reason for this is that, should phenytoin sodium be absorbed first, leading to premature cardiac arrest before pentobarbital-induced unconsciousness, the animal may feel the distress of heart attack. According to the 2020 American Veterinary Medical Association euthanasia guidelines, only pure barbiturates are approved for IP injection in awake animals.[3] IP injections are very common and work on all small animals, including young kittens and puppies. However, it is recommended to avoid this technique in patients weighing more than 50 lbs owing to the length of TTD. In this author's experience, the larger the patient, the longer it takes for them to pass. Shelters in particular use this technique on a daily basis owing to the low level of skill required to perform them and no sedation required for pure sodium pentobarbital administration (**Box 7**).

There are 2 approved sites of IP injection: (1) ventral midline caudal to the umbilicus and (2) low on the right lateral abdomen.[13] One-inch needles of any gauge size are

---

Box 7
Tips for improved IP administration

Awake patients should be handled with a gentle approach

Aim for just right and caudal to the umbilicus in mammals

Draw back on the syringe to test for negative pressure

(Unconscious patients are better suited for IV or intraorgan injections)

acceptable, but in awake patients, smaller gauge needles are recommended to minimize pain. Once through the abdominal wall musculature, negative pressure should be applied to test for proper placement. Negative pressure, without seeing visible fluid entering into the syringe, is a good indication of being in the abdomen. If the patient reacts with pain signs, the needle should be redirected. Euthanasia solution can be delivered at a rate of 1 mL/s. The barbiturate dose is currently set at 3 mL per 10 lbs (4.5 kg).[3]

The patient should be handled with great care, whether awake or unconscious before administration. If awake, after administration into the peritoneal space, the patient should be kept close by for monitoring and distractions minimized. All animals relax smoother into anesthesia when their environment is calm and quiet. As they experience the first stages of anesthesia, the owner may witness paddling, disorientation, lip licking, and even vocalization as the drug takes effect in the brain. Once they are in stage 3 of anesthesia and approaching overdose/death, the patient should be closely monitored for respiratory changes. Breathing is expected to cease well before the heart stops, and auscultation is needed to pronounce them deceased when the time comes.

There has been discussion on the validity of this technique without pre-euthanasia sedation/anesthesia owing to the possibility of abdominal irritation from barbiturate injection. Specifically, a study looking at abdominal irritation in rats after barbiturate injection demonstrated tissue irritation.[14] If subsequent studies demonstrate consistent findings, pre-euthanasia sedation/anesthesia may be required for all IP injections using pure barbiturates. As of 2019, the barbiturate combination product Fatal Plus 3, containing sodium pentobarbital and lidocaine, is being researched as a combination product capable of eliminating the risk of peritoneal discomfort.

ALTERNATIVE ROUTES OF ADMINISTRATION
Oral Administration

In clinical practice, oral delivery of euthanasia solution is very uncommon. It would be reached for when no other methods are available and/or when working with a highly aggressive or fearful patient. Barbiturates are the only drugs used for oral euthanasia in veterinary medicine because of known dosages. The company Vortech Pharmaceuticals in the United States is the only company currently manufacturing sodium pentobarbital in liquid and powder form. Off-label dosing in either form is 3 mL per 10 lbs (4.5 kg); however, increasing the dose should shorten the TTD. According to the American Humane Association's Euthanasia Training Guide, an animal receiving adequate oral dosing of a barbiturate should be in stage 3 of anesthesia within 40 minutes of ingestion and dead within 2 hours.[7] Times vary depending on the overall health of the animal, the rate of absorption, and environmental stimulation. Solution can be mixed with food or delivered directly into the mouth. Euthanasia by oral administration of a barbiturate is very unreliable and the administrator should never assume that death has occurred, even if all of the drug was properly consumed. Beware of regurgitation or vomiting of the drug when other animals are close by (**Fig. 7**).

Intraosseous Injections

Intraosseous refers to the injection of euthanasia solution into the bone marrow space of long bones. It is rarely used, except in the cases of very small mammals, including puppies and kittens, or in instances where a bone marrow needle is already in place when euthanasia becomes warranted. This author could not find conclusive information regarding the appropriate dosing of barbiturates. It seems reasonable to begin with the highest recommended dose for other slower methods like oral and IP (dose of 3 mL per 10 lb) or to affect.

SODIUM PENTOBARBITAL
ORAL DOSAGE CHART FOR EUTHANASIA

WEIGHT		SPECIES	LIQUID	AMOUNT OF POWDER			PRESENTATION		
lbs	kgs	Example	mL	Grains	Mg	grams	5 gr. cap.	Tsp.	Tbs.
1.5	0.68	Kitten (6 wk)	1.0	6	390	0.39	1	1/10	-
2	0.9	Kitten (8 wk)	1.0	6	390	0.39	1	1/10	-
3	1.4	Kitten (12 wk)	1.0	6	390	0.39	1	1/10	-
8	3.6	Cat	3.0	18	1170	1.17	4	¼	-
10	4.5	Puppy (8 wk)	3.0	18	1170	1.17	4	¼	-
15	6.8	Cairn Terrier	4.5	27	1755	1.76	5	½	-
20	9.1	Fox Terrier	6.0	36	2340	2.34	7	½	-
25	11.4	Beagle	7.5	45	2925	2.93	9	¾	¼
30	13.6	Cocker Spaniel	9.0	54	2510	2.51	11	¾	¼
40	18.2	Springer Spaniel	12.0	72	4680	4.68	14	1	1/3
50	22.7	Irish Setter	15.0	90	5850	5.85	18	1 1/2	½
60	27.3	Labrador	18.0	108	7020	7.02	22	1 ½	½
70	31.8	Airedale	21.0	126	8190	8.19	25	2	¾
80	36.4	German Shepard	24.0	144	9360	9.36	29	2	¾
90	40.9	Rottweiler	27.0	162	10530	10.53	32	2 ½	¾
100	45.4	Great Dane	30.0	180	11700	11.70	36	2 ¾	1
150	68.2	Mastif	45.0	270	17550	17.55	54	3 ½	1 ½
200	90.9	St. Bernard (large)	60.0	360	23400	23.40	72	5	2

WEIGHT: 1 kilogram (kgs) equals 2.2 pounds.

SOLUTION: Liquid dosage is calculated on 390 mg/mL or 6 grains per mL.

POWDER: Amount of powder shows grains, milligrams amd grams. For D.E.A. accounting subtract the amount of powder removed from the bottle in grams.

PRESENTATION:
Number of capsules is based on 5 grains per capsule.
Amount per teaspoon is based on 4.5 grains per teaspoon. Note: Use measuring spoons only. Amount per tablespoon is based on 13 grams per tablespoon. Note: Use measuring spoons only.

Fig. 7. Oral sodium pentobarbital dosing chart. Solution dosing based on 390mg/mL or 6 grains per mL. Compiled by Vortech Pharmaceuticals. Oral sodium pentobarbital administration is considered an off-label use by the Food and Drug Administration. (*Courtesy of* Vortech Pharmaceuticals, Dearborn, MI.)

Intrathecal Injections

As of 2019, there are potentially no studies demonstrating the effectiveness of this injection method in small animals. Since at least 2010, it has been performed in preanesthetized equids around the world as an alternative to barbiturate injection in an effort to reduce barbiturate drug contamination of the carcass. The euthanasia agent is 2% lidocaine in liquid form, injected into the spinal column caudal to the skull's foramen magnum and cranial to the atlas (C1 vertebrae), also referred to as the atlanto-occipital space. In equids, the head is tucked and the needle inserted at an angle toward the chin. The spinal needle allows for removal of cerebrospinal fluid and replaces it with lidocaine. The dose in equids is 4 mg/kg. The average size horse requires 60 mL of lidocaine.[15] Although this technique is not currently being used in clinical practice for small animals, it may be an alternative option under anesthesia when other drugs are not available. More study is required to learn proper dosing and effectiveness in dogs, cats, and other species.

Intratumor Injections

There has been some discussion among companion animal euthanasia practitioners of late regarding the viability of using cancerous tumors/masses as a euthanasia injection site. The premise is that tumors may be highly vascular and able to rapidly move euthanasia solution to the brain.[16] Tumors generate from a variety of tissue types in the body, can be highly vascular or not, and may hold necrotic or purulent material. Any given tumor may provide absorption of the drug and another may not. All euthanasia method selection considers the reliability of the method.[3] At present, there is little to no data to show the reliability of this method and other techniques should be attempted first. This being said, if a large vessel is seen entering the tumor, an IV injection may be best. Without data to support a solid dosing recommendation, this author would suggest 3 mL per 10 lbs (4.5kgs).

SUMMARY

The most appropriate route of euthanasia solution administration is the one that best matches the patient's signalment, practitioner skill, and the available supplies. As was discussed in Kathleen Cooney's article, "Historical Perspective of Euthanasia in Veterinary Medicine," in this issue, the practitioner must weigh the situation against the recommended acceptable methods and choose what is best. In the future, as we have seen in the past, new drugs and methods will emerge to drive us forward into modern best practices. Until then, we do the best with what we have and know about animal welfare and the human–animal bond. Our guiding mantra is best set at delivering compassion, confidence, and control along with the gentlest of euthanasia experiences.

DISCLOSURE

Mentioned are multiple enterprises founded by the author. The author is a leader in the industry and, as such, feels it necessary to share information regarding euthanasia trends in modern medicine. The information is not intended to lead to financial gain, but rather impart knowledge to readers.

REFERENCES

1. FDA compliance Policy guide, 650.100 animal drugs for euthanasia. Available at: https://www.fda.gov/regulatory-information/search-fda-guidance-documents/cpg-sec-650100-animal-drugs-euthanasia. Accessed October 30, 2019.
2. Lumb WV. Euthanasia by non-inhalant pharmacologic agents. J Am Vet Med Assoc 1974;165:851–2.
3. Guidelines for the euthanasia of animals. 28, 44, 57. Available at; https://www.avma.org/sites/default/files/2020-01/2020-Euthanasia-Final-1-17-20.pdf. Accessed January 21, 2020.
4. Grier RL, Schaffer CB. Evaluation of intraperitoneal and intrahepatic administration of a euthanasia agent in animal shelter cats. J Am Vet Med Assoc 1990; 197:1611–5.
5. Turner T. Alternative methods of equine euthanasia. 2018 AVMA Humane Endings Symposium and Proceedings. Rosemont, IL, November 2-4, 2018.
6. Cooney K. The growing trend of intraorgan injections in companion animals. 2018 AVMA Humane Endings Symposium and Proceedings. Rosemont, IL, November 2-4, 2018.
7. Fakkema D. Euthanasia by injection training guide. Washington, DC: American Humane Association; 2008. p. 29.
8. Annis JR, Booth NH, Jones LM, et al. Report of the AVMA panel on euthanasia. Ln: council on research report. J Am Vet Med Assoc 1963;142(1):165.

9. Pasquini C, Spurgeon T. Anatomy of domestic animals. 5th edition. Pilot Point (TX): Sudz Publishing; 1992. p. 153.
10. Smith AJ. A guide to technique for intracardiac injection. The companion animal euthanasia training academy. Available at: https://caetainternational.com/a-guide-to-intracardiac-injections-by-dr-aj-smith/. Accessed September 28, 2019.
11. Cooney KA, Chappell J, Callan R, et al. Veterinary euthanasia techniques; a practical guide. Ames (IO): Wiley Blackwell; 2012. p. 100.
12. Coates J, Cooney KA, Leach L, et al. Intrarenal injection of pentobarbital sodium for euthanasia in cats: 131 cases (2010-2011). Presented at the AVMA Humane Endings Symposium, Rosemont, IL. November 2-5, 2014.
13. Rhoades RH. Selecting the injection site. In: The Humane Society of the United States euthanasia training manual. Washington, DC: The Humane Society of the United States; 2002. p. 41–50.
14. Wadham JB, Townsend P, Morton DB. Intraperitoneal injection of sodium pentobarbitone as a method of euthanasia for rodents. ANZCCART News 1997; 10(4):8.
15. Aleman M, Davis E, Williams DC, et al. Electrophysiologic study of a method of euthanasia using intrathecal lidocaine hydrochloride administered during intravenous anesthesia in horses. J Vet Intern Med 2015;29(6):1676–82.
16. Gardner M. Alternate routes of euthanasia. Clinician's brief. 2018. Available at: https://www.cliniciansbrief.com/article/alternate-routes-euthanasia. Accessed September 28, 2019.

Standardization of Data Collection to Document Adverse Events Associated with Euthanasia

Tamara Shearer, DVM, MS

KEYWORDS

- Euthanasia • Adverse euthanasia events • Death and dying • Data collection
- Veterinary/animal euthanasia research

KEY POINTS

- Statistically sophisticated and detailed data regarding the practice of euthanasia are lacking in the veterinary profession.
- Data collection and research about adverse effects associated with euthanasia can provide a platform to disseminate information to the veterinary community and provide reliable information for the public.
- Collection of euthanasia data will help build a better understanding of areas that need further research and may prove invaluable to clinicians seeking to provide better care for their patients.
- Euthanasia studies can be conducted in a practice setting if the investigator is respectful of the pet owner when designing the method of the study.

INTRODUCTION

The formal concept of animal hospice and palliative care is a relatively new field in veterinary medicine, with a history dating back only to the 1990s.[1] Over the years, there have been numerous studies in pain and symptom management but research has been absent in the area of euthanasia and controlling adverse events associated with the euthanasia process. The goal of this article is to review current research pertaining to the euthanasia process and propose concepts to collect and document euthanasia data to support future studies.

Clinical research is important not only to support all participants in the euthanasia process but also to the evolution and advancement of animal hospice and palliative care techniques. It is the veterinarian's responsibility to provide a good death by minimizing the adverse events that may be associated with euthanasia and be knowledgeable about death and dying. Clients who witness a good death are less likely to have

---

Smoky Mountain Integrative Veterinary Clinic, 1054 Haywood Road, Sylva, NC 28779, USA
E-mail address: tshearer5@frontier.com

Vet Clin Small Anim 50 (2020) 561–572
https://doi.org/10.1016/j.cvsm.2019.12.006
0195-5616/20/© 2019 Elsevier Inc. All rights reserved.

complicated grief and emotional trauma. For those veterinarians and staff who perform euthanasia, it also would allow proactive control over the euthanasia process and hopefully minimize the stress for those involved.

Evidence from data that are comprehensive, precise, and detailed allows the profession to evaluate the validity of the results based on facts and to draw conclusions that are based on science. Data collection and research can provide a platform to disseminate information to the veterinary community in addition to serving as a reliable source of information for the public.

Some of the more common adverse events associated with euthanasia and the perimortem period include changes in respiratory rate and pattern, drooling or vomiting, vocalization, involuntary muscle activity, agonal gasps, opisthotonos, urination, and defecation. It is not surprising that these adverse events have been described as troubling by pet owners and veterinary professionals. The American Veterinary Medical Association Guidelines for the Euthanasia of Animals describe "disturbing" events during the euthanasia process.[2] The guidelines state that the release of inhibition of motor activity may be accompanied by vocalization and muscle contractions during loss of consciousness, similar to what is observed during anesthesia. During sedation when the righting reflex has been lost, reflex struggling, vocalization, and convulsions also may occur. They make note in the guidelines that these changes "may be disturbing to observers." The American Animal Hospital Association/International Association for Animal Hospice and Palliative Care 2016 guidelines document unpredictable behavior as a drawback to administration of presedation prior to euthanasia. The inclusion of potentially unsettling side effects in both sets of guidelines is a testament to the need for further research and study.[3]

RESEARCH REVIEW: FREQUENCY OF ADVERSE EVENTS

There are resources available to guide veterinarians through the euthanasia process but currently there is a lack of published studies that attempt to evaluate the frequency of euthanasia adverse events. With the exception of a few studies, minimal published data exist to document the rate of adverse events associated with the euthanasia process. As early as 2000, adverse events were documented in human medical research by Groenewoud and colleagues.[4] Information was documented about clinical problems associated with physician-assisted suicide and euthanasia in human medicine. The authors analyzed data retrospectively from 2 studies, which included a total of 649 cases of euthanasia (535 cases) and physician-assisted suicide (114 cases) in the Netherlands. Adverse events were described, such as difficulty with intravenous catheter placement, myoclonus, vomiting, and prolonged dying times. The study found that 3% of the euthanasia cases had complications with clinical signs, and 6% had longer than expected time until death or failure to induce coma. This study allows the veterinary profession a glimpse into early human research that documents adverse events related to euthanasia.

In 2019, a pilot study of 94 dogs by Marchitelli[5] showed that 52% of dogs euthanized experienced an adverse event. Of this group, 10% had more than 1 event, 31% had a transient increase in respiratory rate, 7% had a persistently elevated respiratory rate, 2% had tremors, and 2% had agonal respirations. A research study submitted to the Center for Veterinary Medicine branch of the Federal Drug Administration evaluating the euthanasia solution, Tributame (embutramide, chloroquine, and lidocaine), documents the adverse events of 81 dogs receiving the drug.[6] This study showed that 36% had an adverse event, with 4.6% experiencing agonal respirations, 9.9% exhibiting vocalization, and 4.9% exhibiting muscle twitching. The remaining percentages were 1.2% each for opisthotonos, anxiety, swallow reflex changes, attempting to stand, front limb extension, and excitability.

A 2019 observational study by Bullock and colleagues[7] compared the adverse events during euthanasia of 436 client-owned dogs that received pentobarbital-phenytoin (PP) or propofol prior to PP. The euthanasia scores were based on the sum of all adverse events for each patient. Examples of adverse events noted in this study included agonal breaths, urination, defecation, vocalization, muscle activity, dysphoria, and intravenous catheter complications. There were 175 (31.5%) adverse events reported between the 2 groups, with the PP-only group reporting 111 (35.2%) events and the PP with propofol group reporting 64 (26.5%) events. In regard to agonal breaths, 9.5% occurred in the PP-only group and 9.7% in the propofol group. Muscle activity occurred in 6% and 14% in the PP-only group and the propofol group, respectively. The study concluded that propofol significantly reduced the incidence of muscle activity ($P = .0079$), but there was no significant difference in agonal breaths, urination, defecation, vocalization, dysphoria, and intravenous catheter–related complications when comparing the groups. There were no significant statistical differences between the composition of the groups in terms of age or weight. Four disadvantages to this study included that it was not randomized or blinded, it was observational, and the dosages were not standardized.

RESEARCH REVIEW: DRUG SELECTION AND ADVERSE EVENTS

Early veterinary research in 1993 by Evans and colleagues[8] involved the study of various concentrations of lidocaine combined with sodium pentobarbital used for euthanasia. This study compared pentobarbital alone and in combination with 1%, 2%, and 3% lidocaine for the euthanasia of dogs, and the purpose was to determine whether lidocaine was synergistic with pentobarbital. In this study, 24 normal dogs were divided into 4 groups. These groups included group A, where the dogs were euthanized with only pentobarbital (86 mg/kg); group B, which used pentobarbital (86 mg/kg) and 1% lidocaine (2.2 mg/kg); group C, which used pentobarbital (86 mg/kg) and 2% lidocaine (4.4 mg/kg); and group 4, which used pentobarbital (86 mg/kg) and 3% lidocaine (6.7 mg/kg). Six variables were measured, including head drop or collapse, onset of apnea, appearance of flat-line electroencephalogram, flat-line or ventricular fibrillation using an electrocardiogram, loss of palpable heartbeat, and loss of femoral pulse. All dogs collapsed within 13 seconds. The study revealed that the dogs euthanized with only pentobarbital had a longer period of time before a flat-lined electrocardiogram was achieved than those in the lidocaine groups, and thus the addition of lidocaine was a reasonable alternative. All dogs in group A (pentobarbital alone) had electrocardiac activity that persisted longer than 10 minutes. Other interesting observations were made during the study. Consistent with the other groups receiving lidocaine, dogs in group D (3% lidocaine with pentobarbital) resulted in stopping cardiac electrical activity in less than 10 minutes but they also experienced muscle fasiculations. There were terminal gasps observed in the dogs in groups A and B but in none of the dogs in groups C and D. Although these findings are helpful, clinically a prolonged is not as troubling as agonal respiration to pet owners.

In 1998, Wetzel and Ramsay[9] collected data comparing 4 intraoral regimens to induce sedation prior to euthanasia in cats. The purpose of this study was to evaluate whether oral medications would be an effective means to sedate cats that are difficult and dangerous to handle. This randomized study had 36 cats that were divided into 4 groups. Group 1 received detomidine, at 0.5 mg/kg; group 2 received ketamine

Table 1
Degree of sedation scale for cats

Score	Observation
1	No effect
2	Impaired gait, slightly ataxic, slightly drowsy
3	Weakness in hindlimbs or severely ataxic
4	Sternally recumbent, unable to stand, returned to sternal when forced lateral
5	Laterally recumbent, unable to right themselves

hydrochloride, at 5 mg/kg; group 3 received detomidine, at 0.5 mg/kg, and ketamine, at 5 mg/kg; and group 4 received detomidine, at 0.5 mg/kg, and ketamine hydrochloride, at 10 mg/kg. Sedation scoring took place at 3-minute intervals for 60 minutes using a scale rating that ranged from 1 to 5, representing no sedation to laterally recumbent and unable to right themselves (**Table 1**). The degree but not the depth of sedation was recorded in this study. Group 4 (detomidine, 0.5 mg/kg and ketamine, 10 mg/kg) received the highest sedation score. Side effects in each group were recorded, which included emesis. Respiratory distress was not observed in any of the cats. Shortcomings of this study included the small number of the cats enrolled in each group, the omission of the depth of sedation from the study, and the absence of statistical analysis.

Another study conducted by Ramsay and Wetzel (1998)[10] evaluated the oral administration of medications to induce sedation prior to euthanasia in dogs. The study was conducted to provide animal shelters options to manage aggressive and hard-to-handle dogs. There were 37 dogs in this randomized study that were divided into 5 groups. The 5 regimens administered to the dogs in 5 different groups included tiletamine-zolazepam, at 20 mg/kg and at 2 mg/kg; acepromazine, at 20 mg/kg and at 2 mg/kg; and pentobarbital, at 63 mg/kg. Similar to their study in cats, a sedation scale that ranged from 1 to 5 was used to evaluate the level of sedation. The interval from oral consumption until lateral recumbency ranged from 30 minutes to 90 minutes for all drug combinations. The study concluded that there was great variability between the time to sedation within groups (**Table 2**). Side effects, such as anxiety, pacing, ataxia, barking, and thrashing, were observed prior to the onset of sedation. They determined that the oral administration of the drugs tiletamine-zolazepam, acepromazine, and pentobarbital most consistently induced profound sedation and lateral recumbency. The researchers described oral tiletamine-zolazepam as producing the least amount of stress during the sedation process. This early study also had a small number of subjects and no statistical analysis and did not officially evaluate the depth of sedation.

Table 2
Degree of sedation scale for dogs

Score	Observation
1	No effect
2	Slightly ataxic, subtle effects
3	Moderately ataxic, reluctant to stand, prefers to sit
4	Sternally recumbent, unable to stand, returned to sternal when forced lateral
5	Laterally recumbent, unable to assume sternal posture

Although oral premedications are used much less commonly than injectable drugs prior to euthanasia, it is important to consider them an option for sedation.

As discussed previously, despite careful selection of drug choice, route of delivery, and rate of administering sedatives and euthanasia drugs, pets still may exhibit adverse events during euthanasia.

RESEARCH REVIEW: METHODS TO AMELIORATE ADVERSE EVENTS

A 2019 study,[11] which was part of this author's master's thesis and published in the February 2020 issue of *American Journal of Traditional Chinese Veterinary Medicine*, is an example of how euthanasia research can be conducted in a private practice environment while maintaining respect for the client. This is a pioneering study because it proposes the use of a noninvasive physical intervention to mitigate euthanasia adverse events (Shearer T, Shaiu DS, Xie H. Mitigation of adverse events associated with euthanasia in dogs using *An-Fa* (pressing) stimulation of acupoint LIV-3 during the euthanasia procedure: a controlled, randomized and blinded study. Submitted for publication). This study is referred to in the rest of this article as the Mitigation of Adverse Events.

The objective of that research study was to determine whether applying pressing using a Chinese Tui-na massage technique called An-fa stimulation at the Liver-3 (LIV-3) acupoint could mitigate adverse events seen during the euthanasia process. Tui-na is a type of Chinese manual therapy that utilizes manipulation of acupoints and meridians to treat disease. The An-fa technique is performed by pressing into a specific acupoint using a firm and gradual increasing pressure over the area.[12]

In this blinded study, 46 adult dogs between the ages of 2 years and 18 years presented to the Smoky Mountain Integrative Veterinary Clinic for euthanasia were randomly divided into control and test groups. All dogs received the same dose and type of premedication and euthanasia solution based on body weight. Five minutes after sedative administration, the test group received unilateral An-fa (pressing) stimulation at LIV-3. The control group received no stimulation. Five adverse event parameters were measured during the euthanasia process that included measurement of (1) cyclic respirations after euthanasia solution, (2) agonal breaths, (3) twitching during the euthanasia process, (4) vocalization, and (5) opisthotonos. In order to collect data, a 0 to 3 scoring system was developed to allow quantification of the events observed. The overall adverse effect score was calculated as the sum of all assessed parameters and was used for testing the study hypothesis.

This study yielded a mean adverse effect score of 1.52 for the control group whereas the test group had a mean score of 0.78 (**Fig. 1**). The test dogs experienced an approximate 51% reduction in adverse effects compared with the control group. Even with this clinical trend, the difference between the control and test groups was not significantly significant ($P = .23$). This is likely due to the large number of animals in both study groups that had no adverse effects. This study provides encouraging results that a noninvasive technique may decrease the frequency of adverse events and encourages the investigation of alternative treatment modalities when managing these events.

These studies used adherence to a general research plan and had an understanding to the challenges of euthanasia studies.

GENERAL STEPS IN CREATING A EUTHANASIA RESEARCH STUDY

Collection of more data about euthanasia from academia and hospice care practices will help build a better understanding of areas that need further research and may

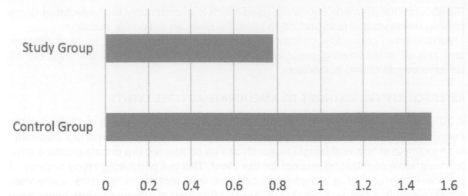

Fig. 1. The mean adverse event score comparing the control group and study group in the Mitigation of Adverse Events study.

prove invaluable to clinicians seeking to provide better care for their patients. Research designs can be selected that are appropriate for the type of research and the researcher's preference. Some common research types amenable to euthanasia studies include basic scientific studies or clinical studies, retrospective studies, study reviews, and case reports. Each type of study has varying degrees of reliability. For example, a randomized, blinded clinical study has greater reliability than clinical observations made from case studies. A retrospective study evaluates data collected from already existing studies to draw a conclusion and also is more reliable than anecdotal reports. Currently, it is difficult to conduct retrospective euthanasia studies because of the lack of published research and standardized protocols.

With the properly designed research study, veterinarians involved with private practice are equally as important as those engaged in academic research in advancing the knowledge regarding euthanasia practices and techniques. Data collection should be encouraged if practical and acceptable to clients. It is of the utmost importance to understand the research process and how to standardize data collection to insure reliable information.

No matter where the study is conducted, the development of a clinical or research question and hypothesis should be chosen based on the need to solve a problem

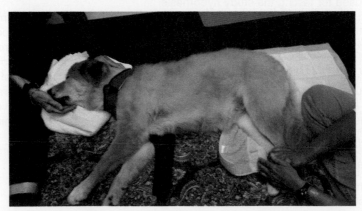

Fig. 2. Photograph of patient in the Mitigation of Adverse Events study with investigator applying pressure to acupoint LIV-3 with the owner at the head of her dog.

Table 3 Example: data collection–medical cause of euthanasia (results of Mitigation of Adverse Events study)				
Euthanasia Cause	Total no. (%)	Control Group (no.)	Study Group (no.)	P value
Neurologic change	20 (43%)	8	12	.373
Neoplastic change	13 (28%)	6	7	1.000
Cardiovascular	4 (8%)	3	1	.608
Renal	4 (8%)	3	1	.608
Musculoskeletal	2 (4%)	1	1	1.000
Dermatologic	1 (2%)	1	0	1.000
Behavioral	1 (2%)	0	1	1.000
Unknown	1 (2%)	1	0	1.000

after completion of a thorough literature review. The literature review serves several purposes because it can discover already existing areas of research and where gaps may exist in the current literature. It also may direct the investigator to other references and provide information to prevent or avoid problems with the proposed research question. After the research question and hypothesis are determined, details of the study design need to be defined; these include subject recruitment, inclusion and exclusion parameters, group assignments, sample size, and the description of the actual procedure. The following exclusion criteria used in the Mitigation of Adverse Events study serve as examples that could be used in other studies. Those exclusions in the study included patients that were moribund and did not require sedation prior to the administration of euthanasia solution, acute trauma cases, clients who prefer to be alone with their dogs during the preeuthanasia sedation period, patients that presented in severe respiratory distress, or patients that had tremors or active seizures.

Randomized and double-blind studies are most desirable because one benefit is that it removes any bias in observation of the outcome results. Randomization can be as simple as drawing slips of paper labeled as either control group or study group from a container.

Collaboration with a statistician helps ensure that the proper methods are used for data collection, data analysis, and outcome measures. They also may help guarantee effective presentation of the data. A good example of the importance of statistics in drawing conclusions is seen in the aforementioned study by Bullock and colleagues.[7] The study concluded that propofol significantly reduced the incidence of muscle activity when given prior to PP ($P = .0079$), but there were no significant differences in the incidence of agonal breaths, urination, defecation, vocalization, dysphoria, or intravenous catheter–related complications when comparing the groups. Age and sex were not statistically relevant. Once euthanasia data is collected, the data and the statistical analysis should be included in the results.

Insights and interpretation about the results should be included in the discussion and conclusion. It is here that comparisons can be made with other studies and suggestions for future studies can be explored regarding euthanasia.

Finally the ultimate goal is to share the research through a scientific publication. Formal sharing of data through presenting research material by way of publication is an efficient way to disseminate reliable information. It is beyond the scope of this article to describe how to write a research article; however, many resources are available. This information can be found for most major medical journals at the beginning of

Table 4
Example: data collection time between sedation and euthanasia (results of Mitigation of Adverse Events study)

Control Subject (no.)	Total Event Score	Minutes Between Sedation and Euthanasia	Study Subject (no.)	Total Event Score	Minutes Between Sedation and Euthanasia
2	3	16	1	1	22
5	2	28	3	3	18
8	3	40	4	1	32
9	0	16	6	1	16
11	8	16	7	2	15
13	5	22	10	6	15
16	3	18	12	2	15
17	8	15	14	1	18
18	3	15	15	3	16
19	0	16	20	0	17
21	1	16	22	0	16
23	4	18	24	0	20
25	1	20	26	0	18
27	1	16	28	2	19
29	1	16	30	2	20
31	1	20	32	1	21
34	2	16	33	1	15
35	2	16	36	2	26
39	1	18	37	0	22
40	0	16	38	1	18
42	1	20	40	1	16
43	5	18	44	3	30
46	0	18	45	0	20

their publications. General manuscript information includes specifics about a publication's review policies, style of text, basic format requirements, overall layout of the various sections, and references format.

CHALLENGES IN CREATING A EUTHANASIA STUDY

Two of the main challenges in conducting euthanasia studies in a clinical setting are, first, to be respectful and sensitive to a client's feelings when obtaining consent for the research, and, second, to put much-needed effort into a study to make sure it does not appear like the euthanasia is part of an experiment. For example, when designing the study, Mitigation of Adverse Events, the acupoint stimulation of LIV-3 was ideal to use, not only because of its physiologic effects but also because it was easy to access and did not interfere with the clients' interaction with their pet. LIV-3 is located between the second and third metatarsal bones proximal to the metatarsophalangeal joint.[13] Applying pressure to LIV-3 and holding of the foot appeared to be soothing and comforting. An assistant, blinded to the groups, was seated in the room behind the investigator so that acupressure being applied to LIV-3 could not be observed but adverse parameters exhibited by study dogs could be monitored and graded (**Fig. 2**).

Box 1
Variables associated with euthanasia studies

Age of patient

Sex of patient

Breed of patient

Health status

Disease process

Sedation protocols

Euthanasia drugs

Rate of delivery of drugs

Route of drugs administration

Besides being mindful of how a study is conducted, it is important to collect as much data as possible for comparisons later in the analysis. Basic data, such as a patient's age, sex, breed, and estimated weight, should be recorded. The author feels that using past weights or a weight estimate is appropriate for euthanasia studies when the pet owner is present because subjecting a patient to being weighed at such a sensitive time is unacceptable. If necessary, an alternative to this is to respectfully weigh the pet after death when the pet owner has left the premises. In addition, the reason for euthanasia and cause of clinical signs should be described. **Table 3** is an example of the collection of data about the medical cause of death in the Mitigation of Adverse Events study. If possible and noninvasive, documenting vital signs can provide additional information. The time any medication is delivered, the time during the process when changes are observed, and the time of death should be recorded (**Table 4**).

Another challenge in collecting euthanasia data is the number of variables that can affect the outcome (**Box 1**). Even if the same drug protocol is used, variation in age, weight, and sex; a patient's disease process; and where a pet is in the disease

---

Box 2
Measurable physical changes associated with the euthanasia process

Heart rate

Respiratory rate

Respiratory pattern (panting, transient increases, Cheyne-Stokes respiration)

Vomiting/nausea (drooling/lip licking)

Myoclonus, twitching, tremors

Vocalization

Dysphoria

Vomiting

Agonal breathing

Defecation

Urination

Box 3
Quantifiable physical changes
Rate of the event–count frequency
Numeral system assigned to varying degrees or magnitude of event
Number of events exceeds a given threshold

trajectory may influence outcomes. The practitioner's preference, selection, and delivery of drugs and the absence of standardized protocols in previous studies make it difficult to compare data. The use of statistical analysis may aid in distinguishing if certain variables are significant. For example, in the Mitigation of Adverse Events

Table 5
Euthanasia adverse events, 0–3 rating system

Score	Cyclic Respirations After Administration of Euthanasia Solution
0	No increase in cyclic respiratory rate (rate remains at baseline)
1	Increased respiratory rate during less than half of the time
2	Increased respiratory rate during more than half of the time
3	Increased respiratory rate during the entire duration until death

Score	Agonal Breaths After Administration of Euthanasia Solution
0	No agonal breathing
1	Opening of mouth hardly noticeable
2	Opening of mouth by half and moderate contraction of diaphragm
3	Full opening of mouth and contraction of diaphragm moves body

Score	Myoclonus/Twitching After Administration of Euthanasia Solution
0	None
1	Twitching/myoclonus during less than half of the time
2	Twitching/myoclonus during more than half of the time
3	Twitching/myoclonus during the entire duration until death

Score	Vocalization Event After Administration of Euthanasia Solution
0	No vocalization
1	Whimpering
2	Moderate tone of vocalization—yip/bark
3	Loud tone with opening of mouth—crying out

Score	Opisthotonic Posturing After Administration of Euthanasia Solution
0	No flexing of neck
1	Mild flexing of neck
2	Moderate flexing of neck
3	Severe flexing of neck

study and in the study comparing the use of PP with or without propofol, the variations in age, weight, sex, and disease process did not have a significant effect on the outcome. Again, statistical analysis allows some clarity when attempting to confirm which variables may affect the outcome.

Any of the common adverse events surrounding the perimortem period could be evaluated in a euthanasia research study (**Box 2**). These items include profound changes in heart rate and evaluation of breathing patterns that are distressful to observe, such as panting, lip blowing, Cheyne-Stokes respiration, and agonal breaths or gasps. In addition, muscle activity, including myoclonus, twitching, fasciculation, spasm, or tremors, could be evaluated. Although more rare, vocalization and opisthotonos also could be monitored. Nausea at the beginning of sedation or release of urine or feces, which often occurs during the euthanasia process, also could be assessed.

Once consideration has been given to which parameters and variables will be associated with the research study, the physical changes associated with euthanasia may be quantified by utilizing various means (**Box 3**). There are 3 common ways to accomplish this. First, the frequency of an event can be recorded. For example, count the number of agonal breaths or cycles of increased respiration. Second, an investigator also could assign a number system to mirror the magnitude of an event. In this case, for example, an agonal breath may rate a 1 if the opening of the mouth is hardly noticeable compared with a rating of 3 if the mouth is fully open and the reflex actually moves the body. **Table 5** is an example of the standardized scale used in the Mitigation of Adverse Events study. A third way to quantify observations is to count the events that exceeds a threshold. In this case, the investigator may count the agonal breaths that exceeds 2 breaths. A threshold also could be set by counting the number of twitches or muscle activity and, likewise, counting the frequency of cyclic respirations that exceeds a specific number.

Proactive thinking about these challenges and application of the ideas presented in this section can serve as a foundation to build future euthanasia research studies. Being able to quantify observations will enhance the reliability of any research.

SUMMARY

The sensitive nature of euthanasia research in a clinical setting is challenging because this experience for a pet owner is a sacred event, and disruption of a euthanasia by the obvious collection of data is not appropriate in most circumstances.

Collection of data in the area of euthanasia can provide valuable insight into being able to provide an improved quality of death and to learn more about the dying process. Alleviating the side effects witnessed at the time of death can provide emotional benefits to pet owners, veterinarians, and staff. In addition to the personal benefits, data collection and research about euthanasia can provide a platform to disseminate information to the veterinary profession and provides reliable information for the public.

Collection of data also will help build a better understanding of areas that need further research and may prove invaluable to clinicians seeking to provide better care for their patients. With the properly designed research study, veterinarians involved with private practice can be equally impactful as those engaged in academic research to the advancement of knowledge surrounding euthanasia and should be encouraged to collect data. No matter what, an understanding of the research process and standardization of data collection is paramount to insuring reliable information.

DISCLOSURE

Author has nothing to disclose.

REFERENCES

1. Marocchino KD. In the shadow of a rainbow: the history of animal hospice. Vet Clin North Am Small Anim Pract 2011;41:447–98.
2. Leary S, Underwood W, Anthony R, et al. AVMA guidelines for the euthanasia of animals: 2013 edition. Available at: https://www.avma.org/KB/Policies/Documents/euthanasia.pdf. Accessed January 12, 2018.
3. IAAHPC/AAHA end-of-life care guidelines for dogs and cats. Available at: https://www.aaha.org/globalassets/02-guidelines/end-of-life-care/2016_aaha_iaahpc_eolc_guidelines.pdf. Accessed September 20, 2019.
4. Groenewoud J, van der Heide A, Onwuteaka B, et al. Clinical problems with the performance of euthanasia and physician-assisted suicide in the Netherlands. N Engl J Med 2000;342:551–6.
5. Marchitelli B. An objective exploration of euthanasia and adverse events. Vet Clin North Am Small Anim Pract 2019;49:554–5.
6. FDA/CVM FOIA NADA file 141-245 Tributame. Available at: https://www.federalregister.gov/documents/2005/06/23/05-12422/implantation-or-injectable-dosage-form-new-animal-drugs-embutramide-chloroquine-and-lidocaine. Accessed August 18, 2019.
7. Bullock J, Lanaux T, Shmalberg J. Comparison of pentobarbital-phenytoin alone vs propofol prior to pentobarbital-phenytoin for euthanasia in 436 client-owned dogs. J Vet Emerg Crit Care (San Antonio) 2019;29:161–5.
8. Evans A, Broadstone R, Stapleton J, et al. Comparison of pentobarbital alone and pentobarbital in combination with lidocaine for euthanasia in dogs. J Am Vet Med Assoc 1993;203:664–6.
9. Wetzel R, Ramsey E. Comparison of four regimens for intraoral administration of medication to induce sedation in cats prior to euthanasia. J Am Vet Med Assoc 1998;213:243–5.
10. Ramsey E, Wetzel R. Comparison of five regimens for oral administration of medication to induce sedation in dogs prior to euthanasia. J Am Vet Med Assoc 1998;213:240–2.
11. Shearer T, Xie H. Mitigation of adverse events associated with euthanasia in dogs using An-Fa (pressing) stimulation of acupoint LIV-3 during the euthanasia procedure: a controlled, randomized and blinded study. American Journal for Traditional Chinese Medicine 2020;115:13–22.
12. Xie H, Ferguson B, Deng X, editors. Application of Tui-na in veterinary medicine, 18-20. 2nd edition. Tianjin (China): Tianjin Jincai Arts Printing Co; 2007. p. 32–5.
13. Xie H, Preast V. Xie's veterinary acupuncture. Ames (IA): Blackwell Publishing; 2007. p. 190.

Factors Contributing to the Decision to Euthanize

Diagnosis, Clinical Signs, and Triggers

Beth Marchitelli, DVM, MS[a], Tamara Shearer, DVM, MS[b],
Nathaniel Cook, DVM, CVA, CVFT, CTPEP[c],*

KEYWORDS

- Euthanasia decision making • Death and dying
- Medical and emotional triggers in decision making • Companion animal euthanasia
- Survey euthanasia decision making

KEY POINTS

- Better understanding factors that lead to the decision to euthanize a pet helps veterinarians support their clients at the end of life.
- Longevity studies are useful in providing information that helps to quantify certain factors contributing to euthanasia.
- Historically pets' appetite has been viewed as a primary influencer in euthanasia decision making.
- A benchmark comprehensive survey for pet families standardizes documentation of family decision making surrounding end of life and euthanasia.

INTRODUCTION

As veterinarians, decision making is at the root of all aspects of practice. Pet owners are also faced with difficult decision-making processes especially when electing euthanasia for their pet. Veterinary practitioners play an important role in helping support pet owners with their decisions on the timing of euthanasia. To improve care for pet owners, there needs to be a better understanding on the veterinarian's behalf on what contributes to and triggers that final decision.

The evaluation of diagnosis, clinical signs, and triggers is not a simple matter. Besides the details of clinical signs associated with the pet's current condition, other complex factors affect the ability to make decisions, making it challenging to identify

[a] 4 Paws Farewell: Mobile Pet Hospice, Palliative Care and Home Euthanasia, Asheville, NC, USA; [b] Smoky Mountain Integrative Veterinary Clinic, 1054 Haywood Road, Sylva, NC 28779, USA; [c] Chicago Veterinary Geriatrics, 1544 West Thorndale Avenue, Unit 1, Chicago, IL 60660, USA
* Corresponding author.
E-mail address: chicagoveterinarygeriatrics@gmail.com

Vet Clin Small Anim 50 (2020) 573–589
https://doi.org/10.1016/j.cvsm.2019.12.007
0195-5616/20/© 2020 Elsevier Inc. All rights reserved.

trends that influence choices. Major factors (other than clinical signs) that influence decision making include past life experiences, cognitive biases, age, socioeconomic status, individual differences in cognitive abilities, one's belief in personal relevance, and escalation in commitment.[1] In addition, psychosocial factors, degree of attachment, representations of death, and perceived veterinary support may also impact euthanasia decision making and bereavement.[2-4] For more details on the significance for various client factors during the euthanasia decision making process, see Mary Beth Spitznagel and colleagues' article, "Euthanasia from the Veterinary Client's Perspective: Psychosocial Contributors to Euthanasia Decision-Making," in this issue.

There are two major reasons to learn more about the dynamics behind euthanasia decision making. First, it guides and identifies areas of concern by the pet owner that lead to the decision of euthanasia. Increased knowledge about clinical signs and triggers that lead to euthanasia may improve the technical and communication skills of the veterinarian to address specific conditions that interfere with quality of life (QOL) or the caretaker's impression of QOL. For example, anorexia and hyporexia are seen by pet owners as common reasons to euthanize (discussed later).

Veterinarians that have an advanced understanding of the role appetite plays as it relates to specific disease processes and at end of life are better able to support the client's concerns. The pet owner should have better peace of mind knowing that important components of care had been thoroughly supported. By focusing on areas of most concern, the veterinarian can provide the best care possible.

Second, it prioritizes various areas to research on symptom management during end of life. More studies are needed, such as the research done by Kathmann and co-workers,[5] which documented the importance of early introduction of physiotherapy to extend ambulation in dogs with degenerative myelopathy. Because mobility is a common physical change associated with increased caretaker burden and is also a common reason to euthanize, spending time addressing research in this area is important. Additional research on the other common triggers to reduce caretaker burden may create a foundation for best practices.

The ultimate diagnosis at the end of life is different than the causes that guide the decision for a pet owner to euthanize. It is important to understand that the cause of death is different from the cause of euthanasia. The following sections discuss observations, conclusions, and insight into clinical signs, diagnosis, and triggers in the decision-making process. Information obtained from longevity data quantifies the leading cause of death for dogs, with several studies stratifying findings based on body mass and breed. Data collected from other studies explore the incidence of anorexia, incontinence, mobility, dementia, and other clinical signs surrounding death. Introduction on how to standardize documentation of family decision-making information surrounding end of life is also discussed. By better understanding the triggers and the clinical signs contributing to euthanasia decision making, practitioners can offer more support to the client and proactively manage symptoms deemed most important to the client. Such information is invaluable in maximizing the quality of care for the patient and the family.

LONGEVITY DATA

Several studies have focused on the cause of death and life expectancy for dogs.[6-18] Fleming and colleagues[16] evaluated 74,556 dogs accounted for in the veterinary medical data base as having died of specific pathophysiologic and organ system-based etiologies (**Fig. 1**). Breed and size (body mass) were evaluated in this

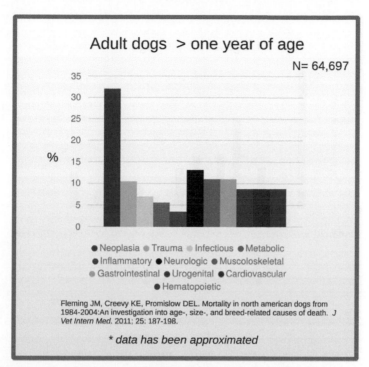

Fig. 1. Fleming and colleagues: cause of death. (*From* Fleming JM, Creevy KE, Promislow DEL. Mortality in North American dogs from 1984-2004: an investigation into age-, size-, and breed-related causes of death. *J Vet Intern Med.* 2011; 25: 187-198.)

context. Findings from this study confirmed increased longevity for smaller breed dogs versus larger breed dogs. Within breeds, larger dogs (body mass) were found to have an increased life span as compared with smaller dogs. This study illustrated the mortality trajectory of specific pathophysiologic etiologies over time. These data are particularly useful because they inform clinical focus and preparation as pets age. Inoue and colleagues[17] examined pet insurance data of 4169 pet dogs owned in Japan who had died.[17] The investigators found the top five causes of death to be neoplasia (622), followed by cardiovascular (380), urogenital (258), digestive (245), and neuromuscular system disorders (208). In this study the investigators combined neurologic diseases with musculoskeletal diseases (**Fig. 2**). This designation may be useful in evaluating older pets, who frequently suffer from impairment in both bodily systems. O'Neill and colleagues[18] evaluated the cause of death for dogs examined at general veterinary practices in England. This study also found neoplasia to be the leading cause of death.

Patient populations, specifically geriatric pets, may have comorbidities making it difficult to determine the primary biologic cause of demise. In addition, diagnoses that are present may be presumptive, confounding precision in categorization. Often times nonbiologic factors (not wanting the pet to suffer) combine with specific clinical signs to prompt a decision to euthanize. The studies described previously are informative in providing a backdrop as to how one conceptualizes how and why pets die. Although data for these studies were obtained from different sources (veterinary referral hospital, pet insurance data, general practice), general trends are evident.

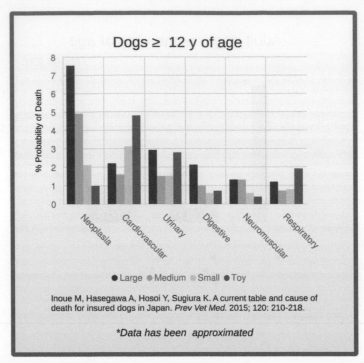

Fig. 2. Inoue and colleagues: cause of death. (*From* Inoue M, Hasegawa A, Hosoi Y, Sugiura K. A current table and cause of death for insured dogs in Japan. *Prev Vet Med.* 2015; 120: 210-218.)

VETERINARY HOSPICE AND PALLIATIVE MEDICINE DATA

The rapid growth of veterinary practices focused exclusively on veterinary hospice and palliative medicine has afforded a patient data set that is new to veterinary medicine. A pilot study conducted by Shearer and Marchitelli compared the primary pathophysiologic process prompting euthanasia in a mobile practice versus a stationary veterinary clinic (**Table 1**). The mobile practice provided palliative, hospice, and home euthanasia services exclusively, whereas the general practice provided physical medicine modalities, traditional Chinese veterinary medicine, and hospice and palliative care. Both practices reported neoplasia as the leading pathophysiologic cause of death. This is similar to those findings reported in the previously mentioned longevity data. Differences were also apparent, because impaired mobility was the second cause of death for dogs and cats in the mobile practice, and the eighth cause of death for dogs who had visited the veterinary clinic. This is somewhat expected because many dogs with impaired mobility may not be able to physically travel to the veterinary clinic for euthanasia. In addition, pets with acute critical illness may be more likely to visit a stationary veterinary practice with the intention of pursuing advanced diagnostics. It is also likely that the physical medicine (manual therapies, laser therapy, extracorporeal shockwave therapy, pulsed signal therapy, pulsed electromagnetic therapy, and hydrotherapy) provided at the stationary clinic slowed the progression of mobility impairment and thus this subset of dogs were more likely to succumb to other disease processes. The greater number of dogs seen by the mobile practice (349) compared with the stationary practice (36) is one drawback of this data set and thus makes these findings

Table 1
Leading cause of death: mobile palliative care/hospice practice versus veterinary clinic

	Mobile Practice N = 349 Dogs			Stationary Veterinary Clinic N = 46 Dogs
Shearer/Marchitelli (2015, unpublished data)				
Neoplasia	127	36.3%	Neoplasia	11	23.9%
Impaired mobility	135	38.6%	Neurologic disease	9	19.5%
Neurologic disease	32	9.1%	Chronic renal failure	7	15.2%
Cognitive dysfunction + mobility	29	8.3%	Congestive heart failure/cardiovascular	7	15.2%
Chronic renal failure	7	2.0%	Gastrointestinal	2	4.3%
Congestive heart failure	7	2.0%			

preliminary in nature. Future studies comparing patients at various types of practices and patient populations will be helpful in delineating overall general trends if such trends are evident.

Clinical signs described as contributing to the decision to euthanize are of primary or secondary importance but nonetheless may have a cumulative effect on decision making. Certain clinical signs may be more prevalent in end-stage disease and may or may not be correlated with specific diagnoses. Such information can help guide clinicians in preferencing the most salient aspects of symptom management in end-stage disease. Understanding the frequency and importance of symptoms with respect to euthanasia decision making can also help clinicians better prepare pet owners for what to expect. A pilot study conducted by Marchitelli from 2018 to 2019 (unpublished data) investigated clinical signs commonly present at the time of euthanasia for dogs and cats. Poor appetite, impaired mobility, incontinence (urinary and/or fecal), confusion, and gastrointestinal signs were the top five clinical signs recorded at the time of euthanasia for 126 dogs seen for in-home euthanasia. Appetite was considered poor if normal dietary intake was decreased (hyporexia), was abnormal (ie, only eating people food/dysrexia), or was absent entirely (anorexia). Other symptoms frequently reported at the time of euthanasia for dogs were altered sleep, weakness, anxiety, and panting (**Fig. 3**).

The top five clinical signs described for 50 cats at the time of euthanasia were poor appetite (decreased or absent), impaired mobility (including unsteady gait), weight loss, weakness, and vomiting (**Fig. 4**).

In this study, poor appetite followed by impaired mobility were the two most frequently recorded clinical signs for dogs and cats. Weight loss was reported more frequently for cats (40.0%) than dogs (11.1%). Both confusion and impaired sleep were reported more commonly for dogs than cats. It is important to recognize that the frequency alone of clinical signs reported at the time of euthanasia may or may not necessarily correlate with their significance and influence on euthanasia decision making. Future studies examining the impact of symptoms on owner's perception of QOL and suffering will provide a more complete understanding of how specific symptoms factor into decision making.

Historically, lack of appetite has been the primary factor driving euthanasia decision making in western culture. This rational is present in the veterinary medical field

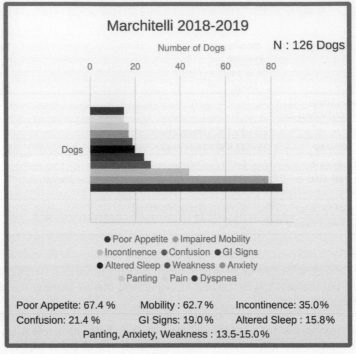

Fig. 3. Clinical signs at the time of euthanasia for 126 dogs. GI, gastrointestinal.

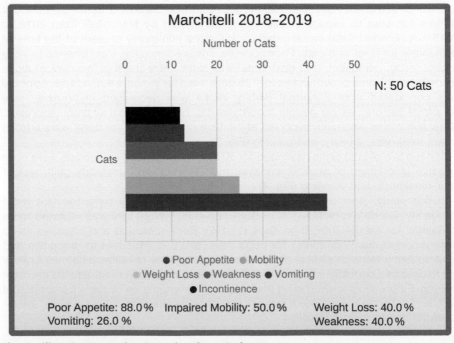

Fig. 4. Clinical signs at the time of euthanasia for 50 cats.

and among lay people. The established gold standard of "when he/she stops eating," although ubiquitous, has not been examined scientifically in the context of QOL evaluation nor as it relates to specific disease states, species, or individual variation. Clinical studies investigating appetite at the time of euthanasia, taking into consideration the factors previously mentioned, may help to shed light on the prevalence of appetite alternations in sick patient populations. Dispelling cultural myths regarding appetite may help pet owners have a more realistic assessment of the biologic circumstances they may find themselves in when their pet becomes sick and QOL is compromised.

Data collected from the pilot study previously described (Marchitelli 2018–2019) observed the appetite of dogs and cats at the time of euthanasia. Appetite was recorded as increased (hyperrexia), decreased (hyporexia), normal, or absent (anorexia) (**Figs. 5** and **6**). Approximately one-third of dogs were eating normally at the time of euthanasia. A total of 67.4% of dogs euthanized had a reduced appetite or had stopped eating entirely. In contrast, 88.0% of cats were not eating at all or had a reduced appetite at the time of euthanasia. Cats who are ill seem to be more vulnerable to fluctuations in appetite. This could be accounted for as a species difference alone, whereas cat's appetite is affected more frequently when they are sick compared with dogs. In addition, cats may be afflicted with diseases that are more likely to cause inappetence, such as chronic renal failure. Inappetence also may be more appreciable in cats, because dogs may be more amenable to temptation as a result of their interest in a wider variety of food items, such as people food when they are not feeling well. Pets lack of interest in food is source of great anxiety for pet owners. Having a better understanding of the number of dogs and cats that are affected in this way, and how appetite is influenced across end-stage disease trajectories, helps pet owners and clinicians address this issue compassionately and effectively.

The context within which pet owners frame their primary reasons for choosing euthanasia at a particular point in time is seen as similar to the conceptual framework human patients apply when choose medical aid in dying. A study by Dees and colleagues[19] examined the reasons patients requested assistance in dying.

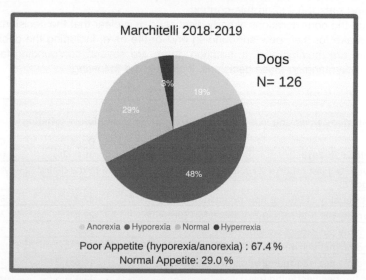

Fig. 5. Appetite at the time of euthanasia for 126 dogs.

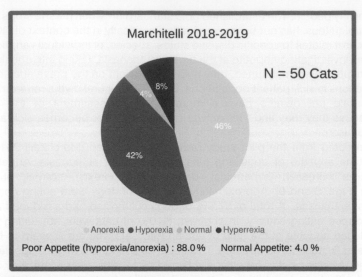

Fig. 6. Appetite at the time of euthanasia for 50 cats.

This study illustrated the importance of time (past, present, and future) in evaluating suffering. The pilot study by Marchitelli 2018 to 2019 also evaluated pet owners' perceptions at the time the decision to euthanize was made. These reasons can also be viewed in terms of past, present, and future suffering (**Table 2**). The categories listed are not mutually exclusive, and it is likely pet owners viewed decision making in terms of their pets' immediate present, and past and future. Such insights are useful in understanding how pet owners view suffering and discomfort and how these factors affect euthanasia decision making. It is interesting to note, although pain was not one of the top five clinical signs observed by pet owners directly for either dogs or cats, concern about pain and suffering is nonetheless of considerable importance for pet owners of dogs (29.4%) and cats (38.0%) in this context.

Based on the considerations already discussed, it is clear that the decisions clients (families) make for their pets surrounding end-of-life care, including the decision for euthanasia, are multifactorial. In addition, there are several confounding factors in terms of understanding these decisions, including the following:

Table 2		
Euthanasia decision making in the context of past, present, and future suffering		
Marchitelli 2018–2019	**Dogs** **(n = l26)**	**Cats** **(n = 50)**
What is your biggest concern for your pet at this time in addition to the clinical signs you have described?		
My pet's quality of life has now declined (present)	42.9%	38.0%
Concern my pet is in pain or has discomfort (present)	29.4%	38.0%
Concern my pet cannot walk (present)	26.2%	38.0%
Worried my pet will get worse (future)	23.8%	30.0%
Worried my pet is suffering/will suffer (present)	16.6%	12.0%
My pet has been declining (past)	11.1%	4.0%

- Full understanding of the patient's health status
  - Lack of any diagnosis/investigation of the pet's health status.
  - Lack of complete diagnosis or staging of known diseases.
- Method of data collection
  - Family reporting of euthanasia triggers: this may leave out details of the pet's formal diagnosis and/or inability to fully describe clinical signs/symptoms that their pet is experiencing.
  - Veterinarian reporting of euthanasia triggers: this may leave out the family's perception of what motivated their decision making. In addition, evaluating pain, anxiety, and many other QOL parameters based on in-clinic presentation may be unreliable because the patient may behave differently at home.

Of these factors, it is generally not possible to control the variables of lack of diagnostic testing and disease staging except in funded and controlled prospective studies (or in the case of retrospective studies, limited patient selection). Therefore, we focus on the variables of family versus veterinarian reporting.

Recent publications, including those already discussed, are starting to give a better understanding of how to name and characterize the factors that may trigger or motivate the decision to pursue euthanasia. These decisions have largely been investigated based on presence of systemic disease (SDZ) conditions and accompanying clinical signs/symptoms that may lead to a reduced QOL, thereby elucidating many important factors from these categories that contribute to the decision for euthanasia. These studies have also provided the understanding that such decisions are not necessarily straightforward or rooted in more simplistic narrow binary parameters, such as eating or not eating.

A retrospective study by Bennett and Cook[20] explored family-reported reasons for euthanasia or death over the course of 1 year. This study described the entire patient population of a mobile practice with services limited to palliative medicine, including in-home euthanasia, for 310 dogs and 84 cats. Based on family responses, reasons for euthanasia/death were described as the following:

- QOL parameters (clinical signs/symptoms):
  - General decline (no specific symptoms described)
  - Loss of mobility
  - Incontinence (urinary and/or fecal)
  - Anorexia
  - Dyspnea
- SDZ parameters (either formally diagnosed or strongly suspected):
  - Neoplasia
  - Organ failure (heart, kidney, liver)
  - Cognitive dysfunction syndrome
  - Other (endocrine, seizures, immune mediated)
  - Behavioral (aggression)

Notable differences were observed in terms of how commonly QOL and SDZ parameters were reported for cats versus dogs in general, and which specific parameters were more common in each species. At least one QOL parameter was reported for 47.6% of cats and for 73.9% of dogs (**Fig. 7**A, B). Therefore, QOL as a trigger was found to be more common in dogs than in cats. In addition, general decline (50%) was by far the most commonly reported clinical sign in cats, whereas loss of mobility (82.5%) was by far the most commonly reported clinical sign in dogs.

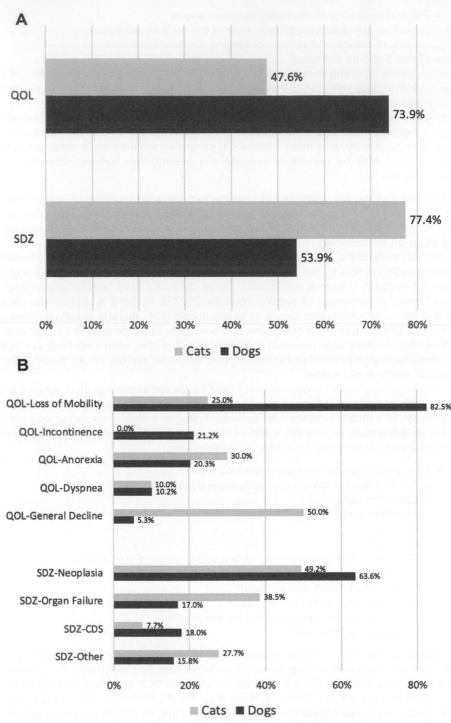

Fig. 7. Reporting of QOL and SDZ overall (a) for cats and dogs and specific QOL and SDZ parameters (b) for cats and dogs (Bennett & Cook,[20] 2019). CDS, cognitive dysfunction syndrome.

In contrast, SDZ parameters as a trigger for euthanasia (as opposed to QOL parameters) were more common in cats than in dogs, where at least one SDZ parameter was reported for 77.4% of cats and for 53.9% of dogs (see **Fig. 7**A, B). The authors hypothesized that this was likely caused in part by the high incidence of chronic kidney disease in cats, but also by the difficulty that families have with understanding their cat's behavior in many cases. In cats, neoplasia (49.2%) and organ failure (38.5%) were most commonly reported by families, and in dogs, neoplasia (63.6%) was most commonly reported. This is consistent with studies discussed already in this article where neoplasia was the most commonly reported cause of euthanasia/death. As a side note, reporting of behavior, meaning dangerous aggression (data not included in **Fig. 7**A, B), as a trigger for euthanasia was reported for only a small number of patients. All of these patients were dogs (n = 9; 2.9% of the dog patient population), most were in the adult age category (2–8 years old; n = 7), and for these patients no other QOL or SDZ parameters were reported.

There was also the notable finding that no client reported pain as a trigger for euthanasia in this study. The authors hypothesized that this is partially because of the family's difficulty in evaluating their pet's pain level, but also because of their hope that their pet was not in pain. Also not reported in this study are additional factors that may contribute to the decision for euthanasia, such as financial considerations and caretaker burden (See Mary Beth Spitznagel and colleagues' article, "Euthanasia from the Veterinary Client's Perspective: Psychosocial Contributors to Euthanasia Decision-Making," in this issue). Bennett and Cook[20] noted that development of a comprehensive survey used to collect data had the potential to help guide families in reporting for more effective and standardized data reporting.

A retrospective study conducted by Gates and colleagues[21] evaluated veterinary medical records for pets (130 cats and 68 dogs) euthanized or presented for aftercare services after unassisted death at a primary care veterinary clinic in Auckland, New Zealand. The investigators summarized the prevalence of diseases, clinical signs, and additional notes recorded by clinic veterinarians in the medical records that may have contributed to decreased QOL and subsequently the decision for euthanasia or cause of death. Based on veterinary records, reasons for euthanasia/death were described as the following:

- QOL parameters (clinical signs/symptoms):
  - Recumbency
  - Lethargy
  - Incontinence
  - Inappetence
  - Dehydration
  - Poor body condition
  - Respiratory impairment
  - Excessive vocalization
  - General decline (nonspecific)
- SDZ parameters:
  - Neoplasia
  - Cardiovascular disease
  - Hepatic disease
  - Renal failure
  - Blindness
  - Deafness
  - Hyperthyroidism

- o Hyperadrenocorticism
- o Diabetes mellitus
- o Degenerative joint disease
- o Obesity
- Additional parameters:
  - o Cost considerations

At least one QOL parameter was reported for 77% of cats and for 69% of dogs (Fig. 8A, B). For cats and dogs, inappetence (cats ~38%, dogs ~28%) and general decline (cats ~40%, dogs ~35%) were the most frequently reported clinical signs. These two clinical signs were reported at similar rates for cats and dogs. A difference between species, however, was that poor body condition was significantly more frequently reported for cats (~27%) than for dogs (~3%). This is likely attributable to the much higher rates of organ failure (see Fig. 8B) reported for cats than for dogs and the slightly higher incidence of inappetence in cats (~38%) versus dogs (~28%), but also might indicate that QOL parameters were underreported for cats versus dogs over the course of care, as was found by Bennett and Cook.[20] Pain was again not included for either species as a clinical sign in this study.

At least one SDZ parameter was reported by Gates and colleagues[21] for 75% of cats and for 51% of dogs (see Fig. 8A, B), consistent with the findings of Bennett and Cook,[20] where SDZ was more commonly reported for cats versus dogs. In cats, cardiovascular disease (~34%), renal failure (~31%), and neoplasia (~27%) were most common, but with significant reporting of hyperthyroidism (~24%) and degenerative joint disease (~20%). In dogs, degenerative joint disease (~32%) and neoplasia (~21%) were the most commonly reported disease parameters. Unlike previous studies mentioned, neoplasia was less commonly reported, with it being the third most common SDZ parameter for cats and the second most common for dogs. Gates and colleagues[21] discussed similar issues to Bennett and Cook[20] in terms of complete reporting of all SDZ/comorbidities present, here citing also the medical coding system used and completeness of medical records.

Comparing the data from Bennett and Cook[20] and Gates and colleagues,[21] it also bears discussing that the patient populations in these two studies were different, almost opposite, in terms of percentages of cat and dog populations included. Bennett and Cook's[20] patient population was approximately 21% cats and approximately 77% dogs, whereas Gates and colleagues[21] patient population was approximately 66% cats and approximately 34% dogs. This is important because although the percentages of cat and dog patients differed, the finding of higher SDZ reporting for cats versus dogs was consistent between the two studies. Bennett and Cook[20] posed the question of whether the lack of reporting of QOL parameters for cats, especially specific parameters, was simply caused by the smaller cat population included; however, this does not seem to be the case in light of the study by Gates and colleagues.[21] What could be concluded, however, is that families again have a difficult time evaluating their cat's QOL, and that with veterinarian reporting, QOL parameters are as likely to be reported for cats as for dogs.

Gates and colleagues[21] also discussed that cost considerations were mentioned for 21.6% of the patient medical records included. This highlights the importance of cost as a parameter that families often consider regarding veterinary care options for their pets. They found that cost was more frequently mentioned during certain months of the year (Fig. 9A). Cost was more frequently reported in November to January (26%) and May to July (23%) versus February to April (17%) and August to October (16%). Gates and colleagues[21] did not differentiate between cats and dogs as far

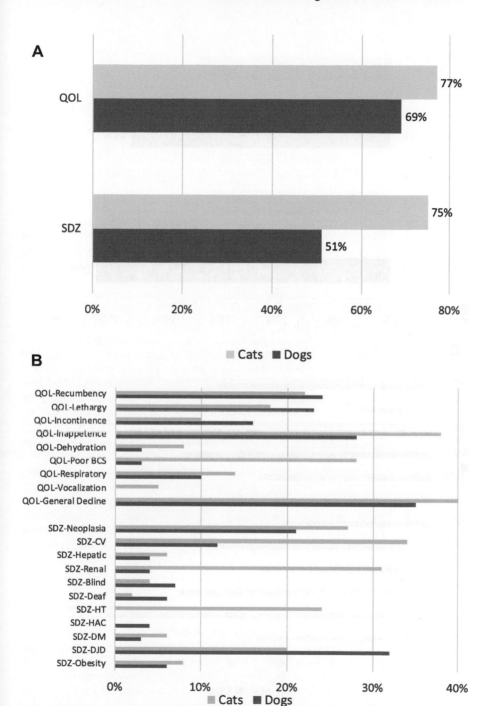

Fig. 8. Reporting of QOL and SDZ overall (a) for cats and dogs and specific QOL and SDZ parameters (b) for cats and dogs (Gates et al,[21] 2017, results have been summarized) BCS, poor body condition; CV, cardiovascular disease; DJD, degenerative joint disease; DM, diabetes mellitus; HAC, hyperadrenocorticism; HT, hyperthyroidism.

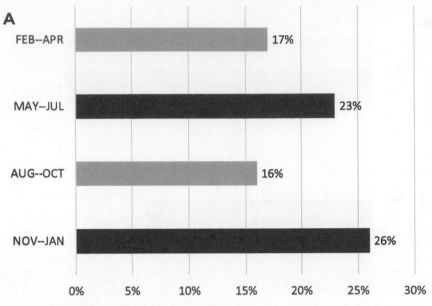

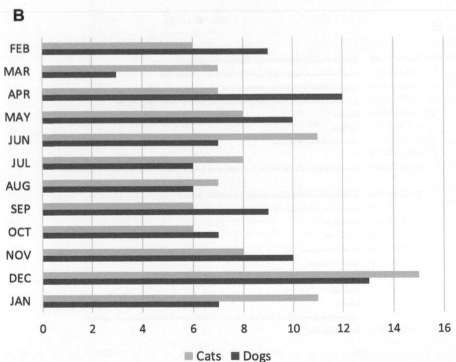

Fig. 9. Frequency of cost consideration reporting (a) for cats and dogs and frequency of deaths by month (b) for cats and dogs (Gates et al,[21] 2017, results have been summarized)

as whether cost was reported more frequently for one species as opposed to the other; however, they did look at frequency of euthanasia or unassisted death by month in each species (**Fig. 9**B). Overall, euthanasia/death was most common in December for both species, with second highest rates in January and June for cats and April for dogs. This finding is likely not surprising to veterinarians because it is commonly observed in animal hospitals that euthanasia is more common in the middle of the year and surrounding the holiday season at the end of the year. These findings highlight that decisions regarding euthanasia are also complicated by psychosocial factors, in this case cost considerations. This brings up the point that psychosocial parameters that were not discussed or included in either of these studies (eg, religious/spiritual beliefs or practices, previous experiences with other pets, caregiver burden) are likely important in decision-making surrounding end-of-life care, including euthanasia.

What is also apparent when comparing **Fig. 9**A and B is that there is a similar trend by time of year in cost consideration reporting and frequency of euthanasia/death. It cannot be concluded from the data presented by Gates and colleagues[21] that cost was the sole reason for the similarities in time of year for increased euthanasia/death and cost consideration reporting. It is also unlikely that QOL or SDZ parameters are responsible. Therefore, we must consider that there are additional factors involved, likely including other psychosocial factors.

From these studies, it is again clear that QOL and SDZ parameters influence decisions for euthanasia, but that a better method of collecting these data is needed. Both studies also indicate that additional factors not studied may come into play, many of them being psychosocial factors. We should also mention the consideration that some animals will deal much better with certain illnesses or symptoms than others. This could be caused by numerous factors, such as response to supportive treatments being more successful for some patients than others, better patient and/or family compliance with care, and that some families overall have a better ability to manage care for their pets than others.

Understanding how families make decisions for end-of-life care for their pets has the potential to help veterinarians and other members of a care team (eg, hospital staff, counselors) understand these triggers and therefore provide better communication, counseling, and options for care. Based on the findings of Bennett and Cook[20] and Gates and colleagues,[21] in addition to further considerations for additional psychosocial parameters, a comprehensive survey was created as a benchmark for surveying families regarding their decision-making surrounding end-of-life care and euthanasia (Appendix 1). The survey was created as an online survey using Survey Monkey software (www.surveymonkey.com) with the goal that it could be easily distributed. This survey could also, if desired, be modified easily into a survey for veterinarians to report similar information for their patients/clients. In the survey, questions were broken up into the following categories:

- Signalment: questions 1–8
- Medical history timeline: questions 9–12 and 18–20
- QOL parameters: questions 30–43
- SZD parameters: question 29
- Psychosocial parameters: questions 13–17 and 21–28

The veterinary medical care team, whether in primary care, or in specialized care, such as hospice and palliative care, is highly valued by families in terms of assisting with important health care decisions, especially in the case of end-of-life decisions, such as euthanasia. It is our hope that in designing this survey, whether used in full or as a guide to what considerations and questions may be most important, that veterinarians and other members of the care team will be better equipped for complex communications with families.

SUMMARY

How veterinarians approach death can have a lasting effect on the client. It is in the best interest of the veterinarian to seek out the most current information on what prompts the client's euthanasia decision to better support their clients at the end of life.

Because of the number of complex factors and the difference in how people make decisions, exploration of triggers behind the choice of euthanasia is in its infancy. Standardized documentation of family decision making surrounding end of life allows important comparisons between practice types and uncovers common denominators in decision making. It was the intention of this article to further inspire investigation of the diagnosis, clinical signs, and triggers that initiates the decision of euthanasia by the pet owner.

DISCLOSURE

Authors have nothing to disclose.

SUPPLEMENTARY DATA

Supplementary data related to this article can be found online at https://doi.org/10.1016/j.cvsm.2019.12.007.

REFERENCES

1. Dietrich C. Decision making: factors that influence decision making, heuristics used, and decision outcomes. Inquiries Journal/Student Pulse 2010;2(2):1–3.
2. Testoni I, De Cataldo L, Ronconi L, et al. Pet loss and representations of death, attachment, depression and euthanasia. Anthrozoos 2017;30(1):135–40. https://doi.org/10.1080/08927936.2017.1270599.
3. Bussolari CJ, Harbarth J, Katz R, et al. The euthanasia decision-making process: a qualitative exploration of bereaved companion animal owners. Bereave Care 2018;37(3):101–8. https://doi.org/10.1080/02682621.2018.1542571.
4. Nogueira Borden LJ, Adams CL, Bonnett BN, et al. Use of the measure of patient-centered communication to analyze euthanasia discussions in companion animal practice. J Am Vet Med Assoc 2010;237(11):1275–87.
5. Kathmann I, Cizinauskas S, Doherr MG, et al. Daily controlled physiotherapy increases survival time in dogs with suspected degenerative myelopathy. J Vet Intern Med 2006;20:927–32.
6. Bronson RT. Variation in age at death of dogs of different sexes and breeds. Am J Vet Res 1982;43:2057–9.
7. Patronek GJ, Waters DJ, Glickman LT. Comparative longevity of pet dogs and humans: implications for gerontology research. J Gerontol A Biol Sci Med Sci 1997;52(3):B171–8.
8. Michell AR. Longevity of British breeds of dog and its relationship with sex, size, cardiovascular variables and disease. Vet Rec 1999;145:625–9.
9. Bonnett BN, Egenvall A, Olson P, et al. Mortality in insured Swedish dogs: rates and causes of death in various breeds. Vet Rec 1997;141:40–4.
10. Reid SW, Peterson MM. Methods of estimating canine longevity. Vet Rec 2000;147:630–1.

11. Proschowsky HF, Rugbjerg H, Ersboll AK, et al. Mortality of purebred and mixed-breed dogs in Denmark. Prev Vet Med 2003;58:63–74.
12. Craig LE. Cause of death in dogs according to breed: a necropsy survey of five breeds. J Am Anim Hosp Assoc 2001;37:438–43.
13. Bonnett BN, Egenvall A, Hedhammar A, et al. Mortality in over 350,000 insured Swedish dogs form 1995-2000: I. Breed-gender-, age- and cause-specific rates. Acta Vet Scand 2005;46:105–20.
14. Egenvall A, Bonnett BN, Hedhammar A, et al. Mortality in over 350,000 insured Swedish dogs form 1995-2000 II. Breed-specific age and survival patters and relative risk for causes of death. Acta Vet Scand 2005;46:121–36.
15. Greer KA, Canterberry SC, Murphy KE. Statistical analysis regarding the effects of height and weight on life span of the domestic dog. Res Vet Sci 2007;82:208–14.
16. Fleming JM, Creevy KE, Promislow DEL. Mortality in North American dogs from 1984-2004: an investigation into age-, size-, and breed-related causes of death. J Vet Intern Med 2011;25:187–98.
17. Inoue M, Hasegawa A, Hosoi Y, et al. A current table and cause of death for insured dogs in Japan. Prev Vet Med 2015;120:210–8.
18. O'Neill DG, Church DB, McGreevy PD, et al. Longevity and mortality of owned dogs in England. Vet J 2013;198:638–43.
19. Dees MK, Vernooij-Dassen MJ, Dekkers WJ, et al. 'Unbearable suffering': a quality study on the perspectives of patients who request assistance in dying. J Med Ethics 2011;37:727–34.
20. Bennett C, Cook N. Palliative care services at home. Vet Clin Small Anim 2019;49:529–51.
21. Gates MC, Hinds HJ, Dale A. Preliminary description of aging cats and dogs presented to a New Zealand first-opinion veterinary clinic at end-of-life. N Z Vet J 2017;65(6):313–7.

FURTHER READING

Johnson LN, Freeman LM. Recognizing describing and managing reduced food intake in dogs and cats. J Am Vet Med Assoc 2017;251(11):1261–6.
Knesl O, Hart BL, Fine AH, et al. Veterinarians and humane endings: when is it the right time to euthanize a companion animal? Front Vet Sci 2017;4:45.
Christiansen SB, Kristensen AT, Sandoe J, et al. Veterinarians' role in clients' decision-making regarding seriously ill companion animal patients. Acta Vet Scand 2016;58:30.
Kiselow M. Private practice oncology: viewpoint on end-of-life decision-making. Vet Clin North Am Small Anim Pract 2019;49(3):519–27.
Heuberger RA, Pierce J. Companion-animal caregiver knowledge attitudes, and beliefs regarding end-of-life care. J Appl Anim Welf Sci 2017;20(4):313–23.
Borden LJN, Adams CL, Bonnett BN, et al. Comparison of veterinarian and standardized client perceptions of communication during euthanasia discussions. J Am Vet Med Assoc 2019;249(9):1073–85.
Ethiek C. A decision framework regarding euthanasia in pets. Tijdschr Diergeneeskd 2010;135(3):106–9.
Van Herten J. Killing of companion animals at all costs?. In: Meijboom FLB, Elsbeth N, Stassen EN, editors. The end of animal life: a start for ethical debate. Wageningen, The Netherlands: Wageningen Academic Publishers; 2016. p. 203–23. https://doi.org/10.3920/978-90-8686-808-7_13.
Meijer E. The good life, the good death: companion animals and euthanasia. Animal Studies Journal 2018;7(1):205–25.

Euthanasia from the Veterinary Client's Perspective

Psychosocial Contributors to Euthanasia Decision Making

Mary Beth Spitznagel, PhD[a],*, Beth Marchitelli, DVM, MS[b],
Mary Gardner, DVM[c], Mark D. Carlson, DVM[d]

KEYWORDS

- Consideration of euthanasia • Euthanasia decision making
- Veterinary client/owner caregiver burden • Anticipatory grief

KEY POINTS

- End-of-life decision making for a companion animal often relies on the veterinarian acting as educator and counselor to the client.
- This study sought to elucidate demographic, human animal interaction, and general psychosocial variables underlying the client's decision making in this context.
- Consideration of euthanasia for an aged or seriously ill companion animal was positively and significantly correlated with caregiver burden, anticipatory grief, depression, stress, and income.
- Only caregiver burden and income predicted consideration of euthanasia above and beyond animal quality of life.
- Results highlight the importance of veterinarians' recognition and understanding of client factors, particularly caregiver burden, in the euthanasia decision-making process.

INTRODUCTION
End-of-Life Decision Making in Veterinary Medicine

Advances in veterinary medicine have made it possible to extend the life of a companion animal, in turn leading to greater complexity in end-of-life decision making. Various

[a] Department of Psychological Sciences, Kent State University, Kent Hall, Kent, OH 44242, USA;
[b] 4 Paws Farewell: Mobile Pet Hospice, Palliative Care and Home Euthanasia, Asheville, NC, USA; [c] Lap of Love, 805 North Federal Highway, Boynton Beach, FL 33458, USA; [d] Stow Kent Animal Hospital, 4559 Kent Road, Kent, OH 44240, USA
* Corresponding author.
E-mail address: mspitzna@kent.edu

Vet Clin Small Anim 50 (2020) 591–605
https://doi.org/10.1016/j.cvsm.2019.12.008
0195-5616/20/© 2019 Elsevier Inc. All rights reserved.
vetsmall.theclinics.com

frameworks have been suggested to aid in this decision,[1] with a balance between animal welfare and client considerations being reflected in American Veterinary Medical Association (AVMA) guidelines.[2] Optimization of decision making in this context has been of recent interest in veterinary medicine, with the field generally accepting that rather than making the decision on the client's behalf, the veterinarian should adopt the role of educator and counselor to the client in this situation.[1,2] Regardless, veterinarian-client communications research demonstrates that veterinarians do not uniformly empower the client to participate in this difficult decision or sufficiently explore client feelings and ideas.[3]

Bereavement and Euthanasia Decision-Making: Different Experiences

It seems intuitive that a client's thoughts, feelings, and experiences would influence his or her decision to euthanize an aged or seriously ill companion animal; however, little prior research has addressed this issue. Efforts to better understand bereavement in pet owners have a decades-long presence in the literature,[4–9] with certain demographic factors such as gender and age, individual differences in human animal interaction factors such as attachment, and psychosocial factors such as guilt all playing clear roles in the client bereavement process. However, these studies focused on the client's experience of companion animal loss.

Client demographic, human animal interaction, and other psychosocial factors may play a similar role in the euthanasia decision-making process, but in contrast to grief, investigations of euthanasia decision making have been limited. In a qualitative study of euthanasia encounters, Morris observed themes of grief (ie, sadness or distress) and guilt (ie, doubt or regret) associated with the euthanasia decision.[10] In a more recent qualitative analysis, Bussolari and colleagues[11] examined the euthanasia decision in a sample of individuals recruited from companion animal loss online resources and support groups. They found 4 themes related to the euthanasia decision: grief without guilt or ambivalence; euthanasia as the appropriate decision, accompanied by guilt and or ambivalence; sole expression of guilt; and veterinarian collaboration with the decision. A small number of participants described their euthanasia decision as financially driven.[11] Cost was also noted in nearly 22% of cases in a retrospective chart review study examining factors involved in a decision for euthanasia.[12]

Although these explorations of the euthanasia decision provide important information, they might miss elements contributing to the actual decision-making process. Retrospective chart review may underestimate the importance of cost because of failure of the clinician to document this issue and/or reluctance on the part of the owner to convey concern over cost.[12] Examination during the euthanasia encounter[10] addresses issues in that moment, but does not necessarily reflect the process leading up to the decision. Conducting an interview after the loss of an animal may be confounded, as well; memory is fallible, and emotional states influence memory for past events.[13] Because grief reactions to companion animal loss can have significant emotional impact,[4,5,14] recall for experiences affecting the euthanasia decision could be inaccurate when investigated after the fact. A real-time (ie, while the companion animal is aged or ill, but still alive) exploration of contributors to the euthanasia decision-making process may provide new insight.

Potential Client-Related Contributors to Euthanasia Decision-Making

Beyond the companion animal's presentation, several potential client-based contributors to the euthanasia decision should be considered. Strong emotional experiences are present during this end-of-life period. Anticipatory grief, or grief beginning prior to actual loss and in preparation for the loss to come[15] may be present, but it is not clear how or if it impacts the euthanasia decision. Might anticipatory grief cause a client to hold on longer than the animal's quality of life would suggest is in its best interest? Similarly, could attachment, known to impact grief for a companion animal,[8] contribute to a drawn-out decision-making process? In contrast, recent work suggests a strong likelihood of caregiver burden during this period.[16,17] Could the strain of daily caregiving contribute to an earlier decision to euthanize? Other problems with psychosocial functioning have been demonstrated in owners of a seriously ill companion animal, including elevated levels of depressive symptoms, high stress, and lower quality of life,[16–18] all of which may also impact decision making. In addition to psychosocial and human interaction variables, demographic variables must be considered. Client age[19] and income[20,21] have both shown significant relationships with distress during a companion animal's serious illness. In order to fully appreciate the client's perspective and encourage his or her participation in the euthanasia decision, it is important to understand the interplay of these factors and their potential impact on the client's thought processes.

Current Work

The current study was conducted to examine client-related contributors to the euthanasia decision while the companion animal is still alive. First, the authors developed a measure to quantify steps taken toward the euthanasia decision for an aged or seriously ill companion animal, validating this measure in relation to subsequent euthanasia for that animal. Second, after controlling for the companion animal's presentation, the authors explored contribution of multiple client variables to steps toward a decision to euthanize, including demographic factors (ie, gender, income, and age), factors related to the human-animal interaction with this specific animal (ie, attachment, caregiver burden, and anticipatory grief), and general client psychosocial factors (ie, depression, stress, and quality of life).

MATERIALS AND METHODS

The work described here was conducted and reported in accordance with STROBE – Strengthening the Reporting of Observational Studies in Epidemiology criteria.[22]

Participants

This study took place in 2 stages: criterion validation of a measure developed for the current study to quantify steps a client had taken toward the euthanasia decision for an aged or currently ill companion animal, and examination of the contribution of multiple client variables to reported steps toward the euthanasia decision as quantified by that measure, in relation to the animal's quality of life, including demographic, human animal interaction, and general psychosocial factors. Greater participant detail for each stage is included.

In stage 1, clients of a companion animal hospice, palliative care, and home euthanasia practice completed an item pool for the measure quantifying steps taken toward euthanasia for the companion animal for which they were seeking services. All participants were required to be at least 18 years of age, able to comprehend English, residing with a dog or cat that was a current patient of the previously mentioned service, and agreeing to allow researchers to extract data regarding date of death for the pet from practice records.

In stage 2, participants were recruited from social media (Facebook) followers of a companion animal hospice veterinarian and nationwide veterinary hospice/home euthanasia service (n = 40,691 total followers) for an online study with inclusion criteria of: minimum 18 years of age, able to comprehend English, and indicating that they currently had a cat or dog that was aged, or that they considered to be terminally or chronically ill, living in their home.

Measures

Primary outcome measure

A measure to quantify steps that have been taken by a client toward the euthanasia decision was developed for the current study (See Appendix 1 for final scale). Eight items were included in the original item pool, to be subjected to examination to determine appropriateness for inclusion in the final scale. The measure created for this work was modeled after the Desire to Institutionalize Scale[23] used in human caregiving, but instead of nursing home placement, items assessed the steps a veterinary client has taken toward consideration of euthanasia for his or her companion animal. Participants answer yes/true or no/false for each item. A total score on the final measure (the Consideration of Euthanasia scale or COE scale) is calculated for each caregiver by summing items, with higher scores indicating more steps taken toward the decision to euthanize.

Predictor measures

Predictor measures selected for the current study were chosen based on brevity and evidence of strong psychometric properties (ie, reliability and validity) demonstrated in previous publication.

Companion animal quality-of-life measures In order to allow both dog and cat owners to participate, companion animal quality of life was measured using species-appropriate measures, then standardized to create a single variable across all participants. The 16-item Feline Quality of Life scale (FQLS)[24] was used for cats. The 15-item Canine Health Quality of Life Scale (CHQLS)[25] was used for dogs. Both measures assess a combination of species-relevant healthy behaviors and clinical signs. Each instrument was summed according to published instructions and subsequently standardized by t-score (mean = 50, standard deviation = 10) using sample descriptives. The t-score was used for analyses.

Human-animal interaction measures The primary domains of human animal interaction deemed relevant to the current question were attachment, anticipatory grief, and caregiver burden. To measure attachment, the 23-item Lexington Attachment to Pet Scale (LAPS)[26] was used. Three subscales are included: general attachment (eg, "My pet and I have a very close relationship"), animal rights and welfare (eg, "I believe pets should have the same rights and privileges as family members,") and Person Substituting (eg, "I love my pet, because it never judges me"). Responses were rated on a Likert-type scale, with reverse scoring as indicated. The measure was summed, with higher scores indicating stronger attachment.

To measure anticipatory grief, the 11-item Caregiver Grief Scale (CGS)[27] scale was used. Although developed for use in people, this measure, which focuses on the participant's experience of anticipated loss, was deemed applicable for this population with alteration of items from she/he or her/him to my pet and removal of 1 item ("It burdens me not to be able to talk to him/her anymore"). Responses are provided on a Likert-type scale and summed across 4 scales: emotional pain (eg, "I feel terrific sadness"), relational loss (eg, "I miss so many of the activities we used to share"), absolute loss ("I try to avoid thinking about the fact that I will lose my pet"), and acceptance (eg, "I'm having a hard time accepting that my pet is suffering from this disease").

The Zarit Burden Interview (ZBI),[28] previously adapted for samples of companion animal owners,[16] is an 18-item measure used to assess caregiver burden. Responses are provided on a Likert-type scale and summed. Recent work[29] suggests presence of 3 factors, which were used in the current study: general strain (eg, "Do you feel stressed between caring for your pet and trying to meet other responsibilities for your family or work?"), affective/relational discomfort (eg, "Do you feel angry when you are around your pet?"), and guilt/uncertainty (eg, "Do you feel you should be doing a better job caring for your pet?").

General psychosocial measures The general psychosocial domains viewed as relevant to the current question were the domains that have been shown to be most consistently related to end-of-life distress in companion animal caregivers: stress, quality of life, and symptoms of depression.[16,17,29] The 10-item Perceived Stress Scale (PSS)[30] was used to measure current stress. Example items include "In the last month… How often have you felt nervous and 'stressed'? How often have you found that you could not cope with all the things that you had to do? How often have you been angered because of things that were outside of your control?" The Quality of Life Enjoyment and Satisfaction Questionnaire-Short Form (Q-LES-Q-SF)[31] is a 16-item measure of quality of life that asks the respondent to indicate degree of satisfaction across multiple domains (eg, mood, work, and social life). In the current study, 3 items were omitted. The 20-item Center for Epidemiology Studies Depression scale (CES-D)[32] was used to assess presence of depressive symptoms. Example items include "During the past week… I felt depressed… I could not get going… I had crying spells." Participants rated their experience on a Likert-type scale, and scores for all 3 measures were calculated according to published instructions. Higher scores reflect greater stress, poorer quality of life, and higher symptoms of depression, respectively.

Demographic variables Participant-reported demographic information included participant and companion animal age (continuous, with drop-down response format), participant gender and companion animal species (multiple choice response format: male, female; dog, cat, other), and annual income (multiple choice response format: 1–under $25,000 per year, 2–$25,000–$49,999 per year, 3–50,000–$74,999 per year, 4–$75,000–$100,000 per year, 5–Over $100,000 per year).

Procedure

Study protocols were approved by the Kent State University Institutional Review Board (IRB #19-071). Data for stage 1 were collected between March and July of 2019. Recruitment was conducted via mass email messages to current and new clients of a practice providing companion animal hospice, palliative care, and home euthanasia services. For these participants, the veterinary record of the companion animal for whom services had been requested were examined at 30 days to determine if the animal had been euthanized. Data for stage 2 were collected during April of 2019. A social media post targeting followers of a hospice veterinarian and nationwide companion animal hospice/home euthanasia service was posted twice. For both stages, the message invited potential participants to respond to questions about how providing care for a pet affects the owner, and included a link to an online Qualtrics-based study protocol. After providing consent for the study, the remainder of the protocol opened. As such, only individuals providing consent were enrolled in the study. For both stages, participants were eligible to enter their contact information into a drawing for 1 of 3 $50 gift cards to an online retailer.

Power Analysis

As the authors are aware of no prior work of this nature, sample sizes were targeted with the expectation of a large effect for stage 1 (ie, criterion validation of the COE scale), but powered to detect small-to-medium effect sizes in stage 2. A power analysis indicated that for stage 1, a sample size of N = 29 would be sufficient to detect a large effect size with $\alpha = .05$ and power $(1-\beta) = .08$. For stage 2, power analysis indicated that a minimum of N = 277 would be sufficient to detect a small-to-medium effect size with $\alpha = .05$ and power $(1-\beta) = .08$ for a regression analysis with 12 predictors.[33] Given the online data collection methods and exploratory nature of this work, enrollment of larger than necessary sample sizes were planned to ensure adequate samples with complete data.

Statistical Analyses

Descriptive statistics were first conducted for demographic variables in stage 1. Next, the 8 items in the COE item pool were examined in the stage 1 sample with a plan to remove any items reducing the measure's internal consistency reliability (Kuder-Richardson-20; KR-20). The KR-20 was then used to examine internal consistency of remaining items (henceforth labeled the COE scale). Because of a non-normal distribution of the COE scale, point biserial Spearman rho correlation with presence or absence of euthanasia at 30 days was used to demonstrate criterion validity.

Using stage 2 data, descriptive statistics were first conducted for demographic variables. The COE scale and all primary predictor variables were then examined for normality and deemed appropriate for parametric statistics. Pearson bivariate correlations were examined for primary study variables. Linear regression was considered appropriate using the Durbin-Watson test and examination of residual plots and the variance inflation factor and tolerance for each variable. Hierarchical linear regression analysis first controlled for companion animal variables, including quality of life, age, and species, examining contribution of these factors in a stepwise manner in the first block of the model. A second block used stepwise regression to examine relative contribution of client demographic factors (ie, gender, income, and age), factors related to the human-animal interaction with the companion animal being reported on (ie, attachment, caregiver burden, or anticipatory grief), and general psychosocial factors (ie, depression, stress, and quality of life). Post hoc examination of the relationship between the COE scale and individual subscales of significant predictors was conducted to better inform the nature of existing relationships. The alpha level was set at .05 and Bonferroni correction applied. All statistical analyses were conducted using SPSS Version 26.0 (IBM Corporation, Armonk, New York).

RESULTS
Stage 1

Out of 45 responses received, 30 respondents provided complete data. **Table 1** shows stage 1 demographic and descriptive statistics. Items in the COE item pool were individually examined to determine if internal consistency reliability was enhanced by removal of any item; 2 items were removed for this reason ("I would never consider euthanasia for any pet," and "I would consider euthanasia for a pet under certain circumstances"). Cronbach alpha for the remaining 6 items was then calculated with an internal consistency of $\alpha = 0.77$; these 6 items together are henceforth labeled as the COE scale. **Table 2** shows individual item correlations with the overall COE scale. Spearman rho correlations demonstrated a positive, significant relationship between the COE scale and whether the companion animal had been euthanized in the 30-day period following scale completion ($r_s = 0.70$).

Table 1
Descriptive statistics for demographic information and measures

	Stage 1: Veterinary Clients (N = 30)	Phase 2: Online Sample (N = 345)	COE Scale correlation	
	M/SD or n(%)	M/SD or n(%)	r	P
Demographics				
Client age	56.90/13.70	48.24/11.37	−0.12	.03
Gender (%female)	25 (83%)	333 (96%)	0.03	.57
Income	3.76/1.33	3.62/1.30	0.19	<.001[a]
Animal age	14.00/2.80	13.27/3.41	0.05	.30
Species (% dog)	20 (67%)	233 (67%)	−0.01	.84
Measures				
Consideration of Euthanasia Scale	3.90/1.86	3.13/2.09	—	—
Companion Animal Quality of Life (t-score)	—	50.07/9.96	−0.42	<.001[a]
Zarit Burden Interview—Adapted (total)	—	22.61/9.98	0.32	<.001[a]
General Strain[b]	—	7.48/4.69	0.25	<.001[a]
Affective/Relational Discomfort[b]	—	2.93/2.73	0.20	<.001[a]
Guilt/Uncertainty[b]	—	11.00/4.25	0.31	<.001[a]
Caregiver Grief Scale	—	32.21/7.71	0.22	<.001[a]
Lexington Attachment to Pet Scale	—	58.38/8.87	−0.03	.61
Center for Epidemiologic Studies-Depression	—	19.93/12.38	0.20	<.001[a]
Perceived Stress Scale	—	18.92/6.86	0.15	.01[a]
Quality of Life Enjoyment & Satisfaction	—	42.33/11.53	−0.12	.03

Correlations between primary study variables and COE scale.
[a] Indicates correlation remained significant following Bonferroni correction.
[b] Denotes examination as post hoc correlation (ie, not factor included in the regression model).

Table 2
Corrected item total correlation with Consideration of euthanasia scale

	Item-Total Correlation
I have considered euthanasia for this pet	0.56
I have sometimes felt this pet's quality of life would make euthanasia the best choice	0.49
I have discussed euthanasia of this pet with family or friends	0.45
I have discussed euthanasia of this pet with a veterinarian	0.71
I believe I will likely have this pet euthanized in the near future	0.42
I have taken steps toward euthanizing this pet (eg, scheduled an appointment)	0.52

Stage 2

Out of 483 responses received during the study period, 129 were excluded for missing or insufficient data; 7 were excluded for reporting on an animal that was deceased, and 2 excluded for reporting on a species other than cat or dog. The total analytical sample for stage 2 was 345 participants. **Table 1** shows stage 2 demographic and descriptive statistics. **Table 1** also presents correlations between primary predictor variables and the COE scale; **Table 3** shows the matrix of inter-relationships among all predictor measures. Several variables emerged as significant, although only companion animal quality of life, income, caregiver burden, anticipatory grief, depression, and stress withstood Bonferroni correction.

Hierarchical linear regression examined the ability of client demographic factors, human animal interaction factors, and general client psychosocial factors to predict COE scale score above and beyond contribution of the companion animal factors. In the first step of the model, companion animal quality of life, predicted 18% of the variance in consideration of euthanasia ($R^2 = .18$, $F(1, 343) = 75.33$, $P<.001$); companion animal age and species did not significantly contribute and were removed from the model. In the second step of the model, caregiver burden emerged as the next most significant predictor of consideration of euthanasia, accounting for an additional 4% of the variance ($R^2 = .22$; $\Delta R^2 = .04$, $F(1, 342) = 17.28$, $P<.001$). Post hoc examination of individual factors of caregiver burden demonstrated that all 3 factors (ie, general strain, affective/relational discomfort, and guilt/uncertainty) significantly correlated with COE scale ($P<.001$) (see **Table 1**). Client income accounted for an additional 3% of the variance in consideration of euthanasia ($R^2 = .24$; $\Delta R^2 = .03$, $F(1, 341) = 11.42$, $P = .001$). No other variables (ie, companion animal age or species, client age or gender, companion animal attachment, anticipatory grief, or psychosocial variables of depression, stress, or quality of life) significantly contributed to COE scale score.

DISCUSSION
Interpretation of Findings

The current work developed a measure of client steps taken toward a decision of euthanasia (ie, COE scale), which demonstrated criterion validity through a strong correlation with actual euthanasia within 30 days of scale completion. Using this measure as an estimate of the client's current standing in the euthanasia decision-making process, an exploration of client factors (ie, client demographics, human animal interaction factors, and client psychosocial variables) involved in the euthanasia decision was conducted. Client income, caregiver burden, anticipatory grief, depression, and stress

Table 3
Correlation matrix of client measures in regression model

	1	2	3	4	5	6
1. Companion Animal Quality of Life	—	—	—	—	—	—
2. Zarit Burden Interview—Adapted	−0.32	—	—	—	—	—
3. Caregiver Grief Scale	−0.16	0.37	—	—	—	—
4. Lexington Attachment to Pet Scale	0.15	0.14	0.44	—	—	—
5. Center for Epidemiologic Studies-Depression	−0.14	0.43	0.54	0.38	—	—
6. Perceived Stress Scale	−0.12	0.40	0.47	0.32	0.75	—
7. Quality of Life Enjoyment & Satisfaction	0.16	−0.40	−0.37	−0.30	−0.74	−0.74

were all significantly correlated with consideration of euthanasia; however, after controlling for companion animal variables (most notably, quality of life), only 2 factors remained significant predictors: client caregiver burden and income. Post hoc examination of correlations showed that consideration of euthanasia was significantly and positively related to all 3 factors of caregiver burden (ie, general strain, affective/relational discomfort, and guilt/uncertainty). It also positively correlated with income. These findings warrant further discussion.

Consideration of Euthanasia Scale

Whereas past work has explored client factors involved in euthanasia decision making after companion animal loss,[11] the current work is the first, to the authors' knowledge, to attempt to quantify steps taken toward euthanasia while the decision is being made. Alteration of memory because of emotional states[13] makes it important to consider factors influencing the euthanasia decision-making process while it is ongoing, rather than asking participants to recall their past perceptions of their thoughts and feelings during bereavement. In the current study, participant responses on the COE scale were strongly correlated with the actual euthanasia of the companion animal within 30 days of scale completion, suggesting this scale successfully measured steps the client had taken toward the decision of euthanasia for his or her companion animal. It is noted that in order to capture a large enough sample of individuals in the euthanasia decision-making process (and avoid floor effects on the measure), a sample was drawn from clients of a companion animal hospice, palliative care, and home euthanasia service. Two items related to general willingness to euthanize ("I would never consider euthanasia for any pet," and "I would consider euthanasia for a pet under certain circumstances") were removed from the item pool because they reduced scale reliability. Examination of these items showed that nearly all participants endorsed that they would in general consider euthanasia for a companion animal, making these items less useful for the current sample. However, this same attenuation might not occur in other samples, if clients are less willing to consider euthanasia. If used in future work, it is recommended that the full item pool be re-examined, to determine if the general willingness to euthanize items are more useful in other samples. Regardless, stage 1 demonstrated that the 6-item COE scale could be used as a proxy to measure where a client stands in a current euthanasia decision-making process.

Which Client Factors Predict Consideration of Euthanasia?

In stage 2, client and companion animal demographics, human-animal interaction variables, and client psychosocial variables were explored in relation to euthanasia consideration. Although several factors showed significant correlations–income, caregiver burden, anticipatory grief, depression, and stress–a regression model controlling for companion animal presentation showed that only caregiver burden and income predicted current consideration of euthanasia above and beyond companion animal quality of life. Consideration of euthanasia was positively related to all 3 factors of caregiver burden (ie, general strain, affective/relational discomfort, and guilt/uncertainty).

Predicting consideration of euthanasia: caregiver burden

It is notable that beyond the animal's quality of life, caregiver burden was the strongest predictor of owner consideration of euthanasia. This finding is not inconsistent with the literature in human caregiving, which demonstrates a strong link between burden and wanting to place a family member with dementia in a structured living facility.[34] The burden of caregiving for an aged or seriously ill companion animal may show a similar link suggesting a wish to escape the caregiving experience, in this case, manifested as consideration of euthanasia. However, all 3 factors of caregiver burden were significantly related to consideration of euthanasia. This means that it is not just the strain of caregiving that is linked to this outcome, but also emotional responses, including guilt. This finding is in some ways similar to qualitative results,[11] finding a role of guilt for many clients who had recently euthanized a companion animal. Whether that guilt is experienced because of the consideration of and decision to euthanize versus more generalized caregiver guilt cannot be ascertained from the current cross-sectional sample.

The importance of caregiver burden in this model underscores the value of the veterinarian's understanding of burden. Past studies have shown that client caregiver burden is linked to negative outcomes for both clients and veterinarians. Specifically, poor client psychosocial outcomes including clinically meaningful symptoms of depression, elevated stress and anxiety, and low quality of life[16,17] are related to burden. More recent work demonstrates that client behaviors associated with caregiver burden (eg, excess communication, confrontations, and nonadherence, among others) are in turn related to stress and burnout for the veterinarian via burden transfer.[21] However, to the authors' knowledge, the current work is the first quantitative study that demonstrates the role of caregiver burden in outcomes for the companion animal. Because caregiver burden predicts consideration of euthanasia above and beyond the animal's quality of life, it may well be that burden is a primary factor involved in early euthanasia (ie, euthanizing before the companion animal's quality of life suggests it is necessary).

Predicting consideration of euthanasia: client income

After the companion animal's quality of life and client caregiver burden, household income was the next strongest predictor of whether a client was considering euthanasia. That income would predict desire to euthanize is not surprising. At first glance, it would seem that this should be a negative relationship, with lower income predicting this variable–that individuals who are less able to afford treatment might turn more quickly to euthanasia. In contrast, the current study showed a positive relationship between income and consideration of euthanasia, that is, higher income predicted greater consideration of euthanasia. Not dissimilar, 1 prior qualitative study, with a sample drawn from companion animal loss support group resources, found that only a small number of individuals reported financial issues as a consideration in the decision.[11] However, high levels of attachment in both that and the current study could limit the ability to detect a negative relationship between decision to euthanize and financial strain. A prior chart review study, which likely had a more generalizable sample as it was drawn from a first-opinion clinic, suggested financial strain is involved in the euthanasia decision for many.[12]

The direction of the relationship observed in the current study might be in part a product of sample demographics; on average, participants reported an annual income between $50,000 to 100,000. This suggests a possibility that individuals of greater socioeconomic means view euthanasia in a different light from those of lower means. Work in the human desire to institutionalize literature suggests that caregivers with greater disease knowledge are less likely to view institutionalization as a negative outcome.[34] The current finding might echo that notion. If individuals of higher income have better access to information about their companion animal's condition (eg, more communication and education from a veterinarian), the direction of this finding may be driven by clients who more fully appreciate the eventuality of their companion animal's decline. Unfortunately, this work did not assess client knowledge about the individual companion animal's illness.

Future work should incorporate a larger number of low-income individuals and also seek to assess client disease knowledge to better understand these issues.

Implications for the Veterinarian

Study results highlight the importance of understanding the client's experience in caring for an elderly or sick companion animal. Caregiver burden appears to not just be a cause of strain for the client, but may also play an active role influencing euthanasia decisions. When a client is feeling overwhelmed, it is important to validate his or her experience, both when the client is considering euthanasia and also on an ongoing basis during a companion animal's illness. Two of the authors (MBS, MDC) maintain a companion animal caregiver burden science blog,[35] which gives up-to-date scientific findings on this topic in an easy-to-read format; sharing this resource may normalize such feelings for the client and help him or her feel less alone.

Routine assessment of caregiver burden may also be of benefit. This can be accomplished through conversation about how the client feels caregiving has impacted his or her life (eg, changes in routine, heightened stress in meeting responsibilities, and negative emotional impact such as frustration and guilt). It might be more quickly achieved through administering an assessment tool. An abbreviated (7-item) caregiver burden scale was recently published.[29] In combination with an assessment tool screening for companion animal quality of life,[24,25] use of this brief measure of burden could facilitate discussion of how to balance the animal's condition and the client's resources, including financial, physical, emotional, and time limitations in continuing to care for the companion animal. When the question of euthanasia is raised, in addition to assessing severity and duration of the animal's condition, the client should be empowered with knowledge of all options, and encouraged to identify his or her own criteria for treatment or euthanasia.[36]

However, it is also important to recognize that a significant shift in a client's consideration of euthanasia could be related to a change in burden. For this reason, it is useful to know how caregiver burden might be reduced. Individuals with elevated burden could be referred to an allied mental health provider, such as a veterinary social worker. Particularly if such services are not available, other methods to alleviate burden might be considered. For example, past work has shown a strong link between caregiver burden and self-mastery (ie, sense of capability) as well as reactivity to clinical signs and behavior problems.[37] Providing education about common problems and possible solutions empowers the client to better problem-solve, which might reduce reactivity and enhance self-mastery. Further recommendations for alleviating caregiver burden can be found in prior work.[38] However, the current study also highlights the role of financial strain in the euthanasia decision. Compared with the current work, the previously described chart review study,[12] which found that many clients express concern about cost during appointments leading up to euthanasia, may more closely reflect the nature of the relationship between finances and euthanasia for most companion animal owners. While all options should be provided, the veterinarian should also aim to be nonjudgmentally cognizant of the degree to which a client has the resources to explore issues of caregiver burden and/or treat the companion animal.

Although the intent of the current work was to examine client-based factors, the substantial contribution of companion animal quality of life to consideration of euthanasia is also notable. A recent retrospective chart review[39] showed that 77% of geriatric cats (age 12 and older) and 69% of dogs (age 10 and older) did not receive primary veterinary care in the final 18 months of their lives. Although continued efforts to educate the public about the importance of regular veterinary care are needed, the reality that many owners do not seek routine care in the period prior to end of life must be acknowledged. For this reason, information should be made readily available (eg, links to trusted online resources posted on clinic Web sites) to inform owners about quality of life assessment for their companion animal.

But perhaps most significant, the current work highlights the importance of empathic communication and appreciation of the client's perspective. In this sample, consideration of euthanasia was related to all facets of burden measured: not only the strain of meeting caregiving responsibilities and the negative affective responses to caregiving like anger and frustration, but also guilt and uncertainty. These are the issues that are already in the client's mind when considering the decision to euthanize. American Animal Hospital Association (AAHA)/International Association for Animal Hospice and Palliative Care (IAAHPC) End of Life Guidelines[40] emphasize not only the importance of objective explanation of all options, describing pros and cons in a factual and nonjudgmental manner, and avoiding bias, but also accepting the client's perspective. To this end, understanding the client's experience is essential.

Limitations and Future Directions

Potential limitations of this work are noted. The stage 1 sample was recruited through a single companion animal hospice, palliative care, and home euthanasia practice. This recruitment method was chosen for the high incidence of euthanasia that would allow rapid collection of data from participants who were considering euthanasia. However, some range restriction in COE scale responses occurred in the stage 1 sample, demonstrated by a skewed distribution, with individuals contacting this type of service having almost certainly given some thought to the possibility of euthanasia. Additionally, although meeting the a priori sample size suggested by power analysis, the sample is small and reflects the demographics of the area from which it was recruited, which may not represent all pet owners. Additionally, the stage 2 sample was recruited through social media followers of a nationwide companion animal hospice and home euthanasia service. This method was chosen to maximize sample variability; individuals would presumably be willing to consider euthanasia for their sick pet, but as social media followers, had not necessarily made any contact or other steps toward euthanasia. This is reflected in the lower mean COE scale score in stage 2 compared with stage 1. These issues do not preclude meaningful interpretation of current findings, but suggest some degree of bias may be present in both samples, because they drew from populations of individuals who have an interest in or were currently seeking specialized end-of-life veterinary services. Such individuals may have higher income levels (as mentioned previously) or closer attachment to their companion animal relative to other samples. Indeed, compared with published samples,[26] the average raw score on the LAPS was much higher, suggesting particularly close attachment in the current sample. Additional limitations are acknowledged in the cross-sectional study design, the specific sample demographics (eg, primarily women), the focus on only owners of a cat or dog, and lack of methods capturing cultural or religious viewpoints. Replication in other samples is needed to ensure generalizability of findings.

The limitations identified suggest directions for future work. As noted, study of this issue is needed in samples representing various populations, including varied practice types (eg, general practice or low income clinics). Full psychometric validation, including re-examination of criterion validity, as well as efforts to demonstrate concurrent and discriminant validity and test-retest reliability are recommended for the COE scale. Factors that could not be considered using the current study methods, such as client knowledge about the companion animal's condition, should be investigated for potential contribution to consideration of euthanasia. Similarly, given that culture and religion can impact views on death and euthanasia,[41] future work should aim to incorporate participants of broad backgrounds and consider measurement of variables involved in religious and cultural beliefs regarding end of life.

SUMMARY

The current study aimed to better understand client-related factors involved in a client taking steps toward euthanasia of an aged or seriously ill companion animal. The measure developed for this work, the COE scale, showed a strong relationship with actual euthanasia of the companion animal within 30 days of measure completion in a validation sample. Consideration of euthanasia was in turn most strongly predicted by the companion animal's quality of life. However, after controlling for this variable, caregiver burden and income emerged as the only client factors that significantly contributed to consideration of euthanasia. Results underscore the importance of the veterinarian's understanding and recognition of caregiver burden in the client, and how this issue affects euthanasia decision making.

DISCLOSURE

Authors have nothing to disclose.

REFERENCES

1. Knesl O, Hart BL, Fine AH, et al. Veterinarians and humane endings: when is it the right time to euthanize a companion animal? Front Vet Sci 2017;4:45.
2. Leary S, Underwood W, Anthony R, et al. AVMA guidelines for the euthanasia of Animals. Schaumberg (IL): American Veterinary Medical Association; 2013.
3. Nogueira BLJ, Adams CL, Bonnett BN, et al. Use of the measure of patient-centered communication to analyze euthanasia discussions in companion animal practice. J Am Vet Med Assoc 2010;237.1275-87.
4. Adams CL, Bonnett BN, Meek AH. Predictors of owner response to companion animal death in 177 clients from 14 practices in Ontario. J Am Vet Med Assoc 2000;217:1303-9.
5. Adrian JA, Deliramich AN, Frueh BC. Complicated grief and post-traumatic stress disorder in humans' response to the death of pets/animals. Bull Menninger Clin 2009;73:176-87.
6. Barnard-Nguyen S, Breit M, Anderson KA, et al. Pet loss and grief: identifying at-risk pet owners during the euthanasia process. Anthrozoos 2016;29(3):421-30.
7. McCutcheon KA, Fleming SJ. Grief resulting from euthanasia and natural death of companion animals. OMEGA: Journal of Death and Dying 2000;44:169-88.
8. Testoni I, DeCataldo L, Ronconi L, et al. Pet loss and representations of death, attachment, depression, and euthanasia. Anthrozoos 2017;30:135-48.
9. Wong WC, Lau KCT, Liu LL, et al. Beyond recovery: understanding the postbereavement growth from companion animal loss. OMEGA: Journal of Death and Dying 2017;75(2):103-23.
10. Morris P. Managing pet owners' guilt and grief in veterinary euthanasia encounters. J Contemp Ethnogr 2012;41(3):337-65.
11. Bussolari CJ, Habarth J, Katz R, et al. The euthanasia decision-making process: a qualitative exploration of bereaved companion animal owners. Bereave Care 2018;37(3):101-8.
12. Gates MC, Hinds HJ, Dale A. Preliminary description of aging cats and dogs presented to a New Zealand first-opinion veterinary clinic at end-of-life. N Z Vet J 2017;65(6):313-7.

13. Holland AC, Kensigner EA. Emotion and autobiographical memory. Phys Life Rev 2010;7(1):88–131.
14. Habarth J, Bussolari C, Gomez R, et al. Continuing bonds and psychosocial functioning in a recently bereaved pet loss sample. Anthrozoos 2017;30(4):651–70.
15. Reynolds L, Botha D. Anticipatory grief: its nature, impact, and reasons for contradictory findings. Counselling, Psychotherapy, and Health 2006;2(2):15–26.
16. Spitznagel MB, Jacobson DM, Cox MD, et al. Caregiver burden in owners of a sick companion animal: a cross-sectional observational study. Vet Rec 2017; 181:321.
17. Spitznagel MB, Cox MD, Jacobson DM, et al. Assessment of caregiver burden and associations with psychosocial function, veterinary service use, and factors related to treatment plan adherence among owners of dogs and cats. J Am Vet Med Assoc 2019;254:124–32.
18. Nakano Y, Matsushima M, Nakamori A, et al. Depression and anxiety in pet owners after a diagnosis of cancer in their pets: a cross-sectional study in Japan. BMJ Open 2019;9(2):e024512.
19. Spitznagel MB, Solc M, Chapman K, et al. Caregiver burden in the veterinary dermatology client: comparison to healthy controls and relationship to quality of life. Vet Dermatol 2018. https://doi.org/10.1111/vde.12696.
20. Britton K, Galioto R, Tremont G, et al. Caregiving for a companion animal compared to a family member: burden and positive experiences in caregivers. Front Vet Sci 2018. https://doi.org/10.3389/fvets.2018.00325.
21. Spitznagel MB, Ben-Porath YS, Rishniw M, et al. Development and validation of a Burden Transfer Inventory measure for predicting veterinarian stress related to client behavior. J Am Vet Med Assoc 2019;254:124–32.
22. Von Elm E, Altman DG, Egger M, et al. The strengthening the reporting of observational studies in epidemiology (STROBE) statement: guidelines for reporting observational studies. Lancet 2007;370(9596):1453–7.
23. Morycz RK. Caregiving strain and the desire to institutionalize family members with Alzheimer's disease. Res Aging 1985;7:329–61.
24. Tatlock S, Gober M, Williamson N, et al. Development and preliminary psychometric evaluation of an owner-completed measure of feline quality of life. Vet J 2017;228:22–32.
25. Lavan RP. Development and validation of a survey for quality of life assessment by owners of healthy dogs. Vet J 2013;197(3):578–82.
26. Johnson TP, Garrity TF, Stallones L. Psychometric evaluation of the Lexington attachment to pets scale (LAPS). Anthrozoos 1992;5(3):160–75.
27. Meichsner F, Schinkoethe D, Wilz G. The caregiver grief scale: development, exploratory and confirmatory factor analysis, and validation. Clin Gerontol 2015;39(4). https://doi.org/10.1080/07317115.2015.1121947.
28. Zarit SH, Reever KE, Bach-Peterson J. Relatives of the impaired elderly: correlates of feelings of burden. Gerontologist 1980;20:649–55.
29. Spitznagel MB, Mueller MK, Fraychak T, et al. Validation of an abbreviated instrument to assess veterinary client caregiver burden. J Vet Intern Med 2019. https://doi.org/10.1111/jvim.15508.
30. Cohen S, Kamarck T, Mermelstein R. A global measure of perceived stress. J Health Soc Behav 1983;24:386–96.
31. Endicott J, Nee J, Harrison W, et al. Quality of life enjoyment and satisfaction questionnaire: a new measure. Psychopharmacol Bull 1993;29:321–6.
32. Radloff LS. The CES-D scale: a self-report depression scale for research in the general population. Appl Psychol Meas 1977;1:385–401.

33. Faul F, Erdfelder E, Lang AG, et al. G*Power 3.1: tests for correlation and regression analyses. Behav Res Methods 2009;41(4):1149–60.
34. Spitznagel MB, Tremont G, Davis JD, et al. Psychosocial predictors of dementia caregiver desire to institutionalize: caregiver, care recipient, and family relationship factors. J Geriatr Psychiatry Neurol 2006;19(1):16–20.
35. Spitznagel MB, Carlson MD. What science tells us about helping the distressed pet caregiver. 2019. Available at: https://www.petcaregiverburden.com. Accessed September 15, 2019.
36. Epstein M, Kuehn NF, Landsberg G, et al. AAHA senior care guidelines for dogs and cats. J Am Anim Hosp Assoc 2005;41:81–91.
37. Spitznagel MB, Jacobson DM, Cox MD, et al. Predicting caregiver burden in general veterinary clients: contribution of companion animal clinical signs and behavior problems. Vet J 2018;236:23–30.
38. Spitznagel MB, Carlson MD. Caregiver burden and veterinary client well-being. Vet Clin North Am Small Anim Pract 2019;49:431–44.
39. Gardner M. Caring for the geriatric pet: exploring their unique health care needs and why vets don't see them in-clinic as often as they should. Available at: https://www.veterinarypracticenews.com/caring-for-the-geriatric-pet/. Accessed September 15, 2019.
40. Bishop G, Cooney K, Cox S, et al. AAHA/IAAHPC end-of-life care guidelines. J Am Anim Hosp Assoc 2016;52:341–56.
41. Kogure N, Yamazaki K. Attitudes to animal euthanasia in Japan: a brief review of cultural influences. Anthrozoos 1990;3:151–4.

APPENDIX 1: CONSIDERATION OF EUTHANASIA SCALE

The next few items are very sensitive questions. We realize they may be difficult to answer. Please try to answer each question as honestly as possible.

	Yes/True	No/False
1. (I would never consider euthanasia for ANY pet)*	0	1
2. (I would consider euthanasia for a pet under certain circumstances)*	1	0
3. I have considered euthanasia for this pet	1	0
4. I have sometimes felt this pet's quality of life would make euthanasia the best choice	1	0
5. I have discussed euthanasia of this pet with family or friends	1	0
6. I have discussed euthanasia of this pet with a veterinarian	1	0
7. I believe I will likely have this pet euthanized in the near future	1	0
8. I have taken steps toward euthanizing this pet (eg, scheduled an appointment)	1	0

Note. Items marked with * were not used in current analyses because of their attenuation of the measure's internal consistency. As this attenuation may be due to the nature of the sample used, it is recommended that these 2 items be used and examined for attenuation in future samples.

Communication
Difficult Conversation in Veterinary End-of-Life Care

Mary Lummis, DVM[a],*, Beth Marchitelli, DVM, MS[a],
Tamara Shearer, DVM, MS[b]

KEYWORDS

- Euthanasia communication • Difficult conversations • Decision making
- Goals of care conversations • Critical incident stress management
- Veterinarian and staff health

KEY POINTS

- Increased effective communication between veterinarian and client has been demonstrated to improve client satisfaction with outcomes.
- Models have been developed in human medicine and adapted for use in veterinary medicine to guide conversations involving "breaking bad news" and developing goals of care.
- Adoption of these models requires becoming familiar with the model's components and subsequent practice using the model.
- Several scenarios are presented to demonstrate common situations during euthanasia in an effort to help the practitioner review his/her own communication techniques and to offer ideas on professional and effective responses.
- After critical conversations, communication is necessary for preserving and protecting veterinary staff health.

 Video content accompanies this article at http://www.vetsmall.theclinics.com.

The quality of our communication with our clients as their pet's health diminishes and end of life approaches impacts the quality of care we can provide to the patient and their caregiver[1] which ultimately has consequences for the veterinary client relationship.[2,3]

PROTOCOLS TO GUIDE CONVERSATIONS

Conversations concerning goals of care may begin when the patient presents with potentially life-threatening/life-limiting disease. These conversations continue as

[a] 4 Paws Farewell: Mobile Pet Hospice, Palliative Care and Home Euthanasia, Asheville, NC, USA; [b] Smoky Mountain Integrative Veterinary Clinic, 1054 Haywood Road, Sylva, NC 28779, USA
* Corresponding author.
E-mail address: lummis.mary@gmail.com

Vet Clin Small Anim 50 (2020) 607–616
https://doi.org/10.1016/j.cvsm.2019.12.009   vetsmall.theclinics.com

choices are made concerning diagnostics and treatment and as responses to those choices occur. These mutually understood goals (revisited as often as necessary during the course of the illness) may guide interventions and treatment and provide a reference point if the veterinary patient's condition deteriorates.

Limitations of time and training seem to reduce the frequency of these types of conversations by human physicians and veterinarians.[4–7] The lack of these conversations may result in unwelcome interventions and reduced quality of life for the patient.[8–10]

Having these conversations is a learned skill that requires practice and even coaching.[6,7,11–16] In human medicine, several protocols have been developed to guide conversations that deliver unfavorable news (SPIKES,[17] ABCDE,[18] BREAKS,[18] Serious Illness Conversation Guidelines [SICG][18–25]). These models facilitate discussions that encourage a full exchange of significant information including the important psychosocial elements that profoundly affect outcomes.

The commonalities of these systems viewed in the context of veterinary medicine are as follows:

1. Elicit the owner's understanding of the pet's illness and current state of health.
2. Ask how much the owner wants to know (ie, how much detail and when) about the pet's situation.
3. Give the pertinent information according to what was discovered in point number two.
4. Respond empathetically to the owner's emotional response and include our own reaction to the information.
5. Summarize strategies and review decisions that are made concerning goals and care decisions.

Recently Katherine Goldberg adapted the SICG developed by Ariadne Labs for use by veterinarians.[6] The SICG is notable because it includes specific prompts to elucidate goals of care. This checklist formatted guide seeks to identify the goals of care for animals with serious illnesses and is also of use when discussing quality-of-life concerns with owners. Checklists have been demonstrated to reduce medical error and improve patient outcomes.[26] During end of life conversations, checklists may be instrumental in addressing the key elements that can lead to improved client satisfaction with their pet's outcome and improved job satisfaction for veterinarians and their staff.[2]

The brief guide in **Box 1** serves to outline key points to help facilitate and plan for end-of-life conversations.

SIMULATED REAL-LIFE EXAMPLES

Acronyms, schemas, and guidelines are helpful in developing frameworks for understanding and offer ideas for implementing such tactics into everyday practice. Much work has been done cultivating such knowledge; however, little effort has gone into investigating and fleshing out the most common specific difficult experiences clinicians and staff face in everyday end-of-life practice. The following examples offer simulated real-life experiences of the following scenarios:

1. Family conflict over perceived quality of life for a geriatric dog with impaired mobility and cognitive decline.
2. Emotionally distraught pet owner facing euthanasia of companion animal who has minimal social support.
3. Pet owner expressing significant distress regarding technically difficult euthanasia procedure.
4. Pet owner contemplating implementation of subcutaneous fluids into treatment plan for a geriatric cat with renal failure.

> **Box 1**
> **Key points for end-of-life conversations**
>
> *PREPARE*
>
> Prepare yourself:
> 1. Take care of yourself (physically, emotionally, mentally) to be in the optimal frame of mind for a potentially stressful conversation.[27–29]
> 2. Know your patient's situation as well as you are able. Be conversant with your diagnostic and treatment plan. Be ready to answer questions concerning prognosis (could put in the cancer Web site) and the potential negative impacts any choices may have on your patient and the owner including caregiver burden. Written notes may be helpful.
> 3. Adopt a stance of curiosity and facilitation; avoid assuming responsibility for engineering specific outcomes.
>
> Prepare the physical space:
> Ideally all stakeholders, including you, are seated comfortably with as few interruptions as possible.
>
> *BEGIN*
>
> Introductions (including name and role) with eye contact (especially important at the first meeting and whenever new caregivers are present) to establish and maintain rapport.
>
> Consider using one of the protocols listed previously or a strategy from the scenarios discussed later as a guide for your conversation.
>
> Seek to develop mutual understanding of the owner's goals for their pet, strategies that might achieve those goals, and the opportunity for feelings to be expressed and recognized.
>
> *FINISH*
>
> Thank everyone for their participation, document decisions made, and implement action items. Provide appropriate resources (quality of life scales, mental health care resources, aftercare information).

Several of these examples have accompanying videos that illustrate the challenges of real-life interaction, particularly in the pet owners' home as opposed to the clinical setting. These videos are not meant to be gold standards of veterinary communication in these particular instances. Rather, they are to inspire future discussion and debate as to best practices in these common clinical scenarios.

Scenario One: Family Conflict

Mr and Mrs Goodman have scheduled a quality-of-life evaluation for their 13-year-old dog, Honey. Honey has severe debilitating osteoarthritis and nighttime waking thought to be a result of cognitive decline, or pain and discomfort, or a combination of these. Mr Goodman believes Honey's quality of life is compromised at this time. Mrs Goodman believes Honey is experiencing what is expected and normal for an older dog and that her quality of life is acceptable at this time. She has agreed to the evaluation for Honey to please her husband but feels it is not necessary, stating to the veterinarian several times, "I am not really sure why you are here." She expresses dismay about euthanizing Honey on the sole basis of her mobility, stating, "Would you kill your dog just because she could not walk?". Family conflict originating from opposing viewpoints, desires, and emotions are common occurrences during end-of-life.[27–29] Further understanding and anticipating family conflict better prepares practitioners to provide quality communication and care (**Fig. 1**, Video 1).

In this interaction the veterinarian maintains a neutral stance while affirming both partners' different points of view regarding Honey's overall quality of life. Mrs Goodman is overtly hostile at times. The veterinarian maintains a firm position of

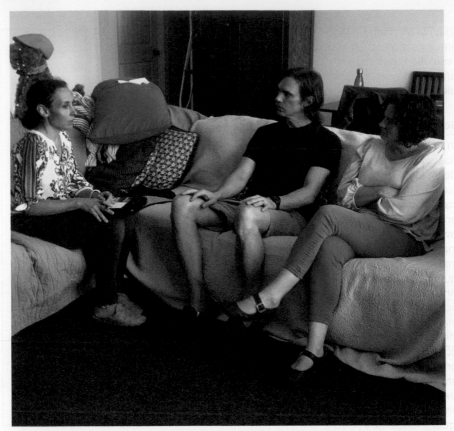

Fig. 1. Mr and Mrs Goodman discuss quality of life for their dog Honey with a veterinarian in their home. (*Courtesy of* 4 Paws Farewell Asheville, NC.)

compassionate neutrality. Rather than reflecting back Mrs Goodman's emotional state (a technique known as mirroring), such as: "It seems like you are angry and upset about having this quality of life consultation and our inability to cure Honey's arthritis," the veterinarian instead focuses on Honey, from Honey's point of view. Although emotional mirroring is not inappropriate in this setting, it is helpful to have clinical judgment and flexibility because each situation is unique. In this particular situation, the veterinarian wanted to avoid the risk of hindering forward momentum in the consultation by focusing narrowly on Mrs Goodman's emotional state. Instead, the veterinarian asked "Mr and Mrs Goodman, would each of you be willing to tell me in your own words, if Honey were to speak verbally about her life and what she is experiencing, what would she tell us?". Although Mrs Goodman is resistant, this question allows her to reflect on Honey's perspective, sense of autonomy, and how Honey is experiencing her life at this moment. Mrs Goodman's point of view is respected and heard on all accounts. The veterinarian also attempts to be relatable in expressing her own experience with her elderly pet with similar impairments and the accompanying emotional struggles she had with end-of-life decision making. The veterinarian presents important information, "Honey's nighttime waking could be a sign of anxiety/pain or both" in a way that is neutral and nonthreatening. The veterinarian also intercedes when Mr and Mrs Goodman are attempting to "one up" each other with a correspondingly equal or superior bad or good fact about Honey's quality of life. Importantly, the veterinarian is sure to convey that the goal of the consultation is not to have Mr and Mrs Goodman agree with one another, but rather to establish a baseline for each of them regarding Honey's quality of life. As in real life, there is not a true resolution, but instead resources are provided (quality of life scales/recording good and bad days/caregiver burden/mental health resources) for both partners to consider along with a template for more open communication moving forward.

Scenario Two: Emotionally Distressed Pet Owner

In this interaction, the pet owner is outwardly emotionally distraught during the euthanasia appointment, experiencing periods of hyperventilation, and extreme emotional distress. In the dialogue between the pet owner and the veterinarian, the veterinarian exhibits compassion and understanding while at the same time guides the owner to a calmer emotional state. The physical act of offering water and a cold wash cloth, while encouraging the owner to breathe in a slow manner, uses physical aids to bring the owner back to the present experience, while providing a sense of comfort. The veterinarian continually reassures the client that she is making the right decision. The veterinarian also redirects the client from her deeply distressing feelings by eliciting questions about positive experiences the pet has had in the past (How did you get Angel? Does Angel like other dogs? What was her personality like when she was young?).[30] This is not meant to avoid allowing the owner to express distressing feelings, but is used to frame the euthanasia as a way of honoring all aspects of Angel's life. In this way, the owner's emotional pain is heard and validated and the client is comforted by focusing on honoring the pet's life. In such cases, if at any point the practitioner believes that the client is in danger of self-harm as a result of extreme emotional distress, such measures as postponing the appointment and placing the owner in immediate touch with mental health professionals should be taken. Following end-of-life appointments, it is important to provide pet owners with resources, such as local mental health care providers and pet loss support groups, in written form. Emotional distress may be so great that accessing resources on a professional Web site could be overwhelming. Providing written material is most helpful especially for those owners who do not have access to a computer (**Fig. 2**, Video 2).

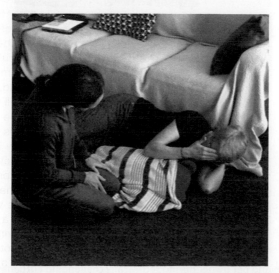

Fig. 2. Mrs Finch and her pet Angel. (*Courtesy of* 4 Paws Farewell Asheville, NC.)

Scenario Three: Emotional Distress Over Technically Challenging Euthanasia

The pet owner in this interaction is distraught by the technical challenges that are encountered during the euthanasia appointment. The pet owner expresses distress and anxiety about the difficulty the clinician has in placing an intravenous (IV) catheter and the extended length of time to death for the pet. In this encounter, the veterinarian validates the owner's feelings of dismay, expresses compassion, and also redirects the pet owner to comforting the pet. In such instances, full concentration is needed to perform technically challenging procedures. This is thwarted by unintentional repeated interruption from the pet owner. To address this, the clinician reassures the pet owner that the pet will indeed have a peaceful passing. She also elicits the owner's help by instructing, "Let's work together. You continue to comfort and talk to Nala and I am going to give my full concentration to placing the IV catheter because it requires my full attention." Additionally, the veterinarian reassures the client by conveying the message that even if placing the IV on the second try is unsuccessful, the pet will still experience a peaceful passing via an intraperitoneal injection. It is important to determine when to move straight to an alternative route of administration to allay the owner's fears and distress at multiple attempts at IV catheter placement. Although in some cases it may be appropriate to try a second or third limb for IV access, in other situations, the clinician should move swiftly to an alternative method of administration (discussed in Kathleen Cooney's article, "Common and Alternative Routes of Euthanasia Solution Administration," elsewhere in this issue). Continued attempts to place an IV catheter might amplify the owner's distress and anxiety. Clinical judgment is required to evaluate the emotional climate of each interaction and proceed accordingly. Once administration of euthanasia solution has been successful, eliciting information about the pet's personality and past experiences can serve to honor the pet during this time. Continued emotional distress and discomfort by the pet owner at this juncture should be met with compassion and a calm demeanor. Medically detailed explanations of the challenge of catheter placement (low blood pressure, geriatric pet) may be less helpful than focusing on the pet's past life experiences and interactions (**Fig. 3**, Video 3).

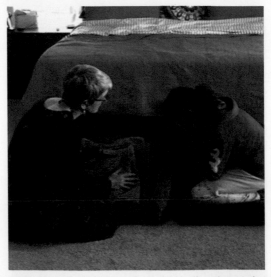

Fig. 3. Veterinarian and pet owner during technically challenging euthanasia. (*Courtesy of* 4 Paws Farewell Asheville, NC.)

Scenario Four: Implementing Additional Treatment for a Geriatric Pet

A decisional balance sheet in the context of end-of-life decision making may help to define various components contributing to complex decision making. Having abstract thoughts and feelings expressed and categorized in written form may help clients work through difficult decisions in a way that verbal interaction cannot. Having a pictorial representation of emotionally charged ethical dilemmas may help solidify important points and facilitate less burdened decision making.[31] It also allows participants to feel confident that all aspects of a difficult decision have been considered. The following is a case example implementing a decisional balance sheet.

Mrs Peak is the owner of Foxy, an 18-year-old female spayed domestic short hair with a history of severe renal disease. Foxy is not eating and her quality of life has deteriorated. Mrs Peak is considering euthanasia at this time versus the implementation of subcutaneous fluid administration. Mrs Peak is considering subcutaneous fluid therapy at home to see if this can help Foxy to feel better for some time and thus extend her life.

The decisional balance sheet depicted in **Table 1** outlines the case described previously. Advantages and disadvantages are displayed in the context of choosing and not choosing to implement subcutaneous fluids for Foxy. Discussing the table with Mrs Peak may help with decision making and prompt further dialogue. Decisional balance sheets are used to explore treatment interventions, euthanasia decision making, and other crossroads encountered during end of life.

AFTER THE END-OF-LIFE CONVERSATION: FOR VETERINARIANS AND THEIR STAFF

A commonly overlooked aspect of providing good communication and being able to engage in serious conversation is to recognize that the veterinary care team needs skills to preserve their own mental and physical health. It is beyond the scope of this article to provide a detailed discussion on how to support the professional's self-care. Instead we refer the reader to the article by Dr Azaria Akashi, a psychologist, entitled, "Ten Tips for Veterinarians Dealing with Terminally Ill Patients."[32] These tips include nurturing one's physical health and mental health, recognizing signs of emotional distress, and understanding personal ethics.

Table 1
Decisional balance sheet for implementing subcutaneous fluids

	Introducing Subcutaneous Fluids	Not Introducing Subcutaneous Fluids
Advantages	Foxy may feel much better and will start eating. Foxy may be able to enjoy her life/ Mrs Peak will be able to enjoy her for longer.	Foxy will not have to undergo the stress of handling for subcutaneous fluids. End-of-life choices will be clear without having her improve temporarily, only to feel unwell again after fluids (will be able to avoid emotional roller coaster).
Disadvantages	Increased stress for Foxy and Mrs Peak as a result of fluid administration. Increased financial cost of fluids/ nursing care. Improvement in her overall quality may be transient, leading to a false sense of hope.	Living with the regret that fluids may have helped Foxy feel better. Fluids may have helped Foxy live longer.

Another tool in veterinary medicine that uses communication to support the veterinary team is Critical Incident Stress Management (CISM). This concept, first used in disaster management, has also been adopted by other professional groups including the American Association of Nurse Anesthetists to help cope with loss.[33] CISM was developed to offset negative consequences of traumatic events. This author (Shearer) has used and modified CISM for many situations encountered in veterinary medicine. Some examples of critical incidences in the veterinary profession include anesthetic death, euthanasia, noncompliance by the pet owner, and financial constraints that negatively affect treatment choices and outcome.

CISM distinguishes between two participants of the incident, the first victim and the second victim. The first victim would be the clients with the pet (in human medicine this would be the patient) that are directly impacted by an adverse event. The second victim would be the health care provider (veterinarian and staff) who becomes traumatized by taking on the burden of a dying or ill patient. Most focus is put on the support of the first victims but the second victims may require the same support. Over time, these traumatic events may exhaust one's usual coping mechanisms resulting in distress and loss of adaptive functioning.[34]

The object of CISM is to maintain or restore the individuals involved to their state of health before the event by alleviating the severe effects of traumatic stress. CISM uses three steps that focus on stress management, defusing, and debriefing through shared conversation with the involved staff.[33] The process of CISM includes providing appropriate emotional support and aims to achieve better mental health of the group postincident, improving job retention, and increasing productivity.[33]

SUMMARY

This article demonstrates how good communication sets the foundation to provide superior comprehensive care especially during the stressful time surrounding end of life. During this sensitive time for a patient and the family, the stakes are high because there are no "do overs" and because end-of-life conversations may exact a heightened emotional toll on all participants. The videos in this article offer a glimpse into a few situations encountered by veterinarians. Each end-of-life conversation is as unique as the constellation of the specific patient, client, and veterinary staff involved. The veterinarian's personality, experience, and communication skills highly influence whether end-of-life conversations occur and how these potentially difficult conversations unfold. Experts in communication have developed recommendations to help support and guide the veterinarian when faced with end-of-life consultations, which may involve challenging medical and psychosocial elements. Improved communication effectiveness requires a knowledge of available communication protocols, implementation of the protocols, refining the essential skills through practice, and embracing what fits each unique family's goals or situation.

DISCLOSURE

The authors have nothing to disclose.

SUPPLEMENTARY DATA

Supplementary data related to this article can be found online at https://doi.org/10.1016/j.cvsm.2019.12.009.

REFERENCES

1. La Jeunesse C. Compassion fatigue: continuing to give when the well runs dry. 2012. Available at: https://www.cliniciansbrief.com/article/compassion-fatigue-continuing-give-when-well-runs-dry. Accessed October 1, 2019.
2. Nogueira Borden LJ, Adams CL, Bonnett BN, et al. Comparison of veterinarian and standardized client perceptions of communication during euthanasia discussions. J Am Vet Med Assoc 2019;254(9):1077–85.
3. Coe JB, Adams CL, Bonnett BN, et al. A focus group study of veterinarians' and pet owners' perceptions of veterinary communication in companion animal practice. J Am Vet Med Assoc 2008;233(7):1072–80.
4. Ganguli I, Chittenden E, Jackson V, et al. Survey on clinician perceptions and practices regarding goals of care conversations. J Palliat Med 2016;19(11):1215–7.
5. You JJ, Downar J, Fowler RA, et al. Barriers to goals of care discussions with seriously ill hospitalized patients and their families: a multicenter survey of clinicians. JAMA Intern Med 2015;175:549–56.
6. Goldberg KJ. Goals of care development and use of the serious illness conversation guide. Vet Clin Small Anim 2019;49:399–415.
7. Shaw JR, Lagoni L. End-of-life communication in veterinary medicine: delivering bad news and euthanasia decision making. Vet Clin Small Anim 2017;37:95–108.
8. Liebert M. Easing the difficult journeys. J Palliat Med 2006;9(4):835–7.
9. Travis SS, Moore S, Larsen PD, et al. Clinical indicators of treatment futility imminent terminal decline as discussed by multidisciplinary teams in long-term care. Am J Hosp Palliat Care 2005;22(3):204–10.
10. Schnittke N. Palliative care in the emergency department: a practical overview of why and how 2016. Available at: http://www.emdocs.net/palliative-care-in-the-emergency-department-a-practical-overview-of-why-and-how/. Accessed October 1, 2019.
11. Vital Talk. Available at: https://www.vitaltalk.org/resources/. Accessed October 1, 2019.
12. Stone D, Patton B, Heen SA. Difficult conversations. New York: Penguin Putnam Inc.; 1999.
13. Wittenberg E, Ferrell BR, Goldsmith, et al. Textbook of palliative care communication. New York: Oxford University Press; 2016.
14. Hunter L, Shaw JR. How to help clients angry with grief. Clinician's Brief; 2015. Available at: https://www.cliniciansbrief.com/article/how-help-clients-angry-grief. Accessed October 1, 2019.
15. Hunter LJ, Shaw JR. Addressing the angry client: empathize and apologize. Clinician's Brief; 2013. Available at: https://www.cliniciansbrief.com/article/addressing-angry-client-empathize-apologize. Accessed October 1, 2019.
16. Christiansen SB, Kristensen AT, Lassen J, et al. Veterinarians' role in clients' decision-making regarding seriously ill companion animal patients. Acta Vet Scand 2016;58(30):1–14.
17. Baile WF, Buckman R, Lenzi R, et al. SPIKES-A six-step protocol of delivering bad news: application to the patient with cancer. Oncologist 2000;5(4):302–11.
18. Narayanan V, Bista B, Koshy C. 'Breaks' protocol for breaking bad news. Indian J Palliat Care 2010;16(2):61–5.
19. Childers JW, Back AL, Tulsky JA. REMAP: a framework for goals of care conversations. J Oncol Pract 2017;13(10):e844–50.

20. Bekelman DB, Johnson-Koenke R, Ahluwalia SC, et al. Development and feasibility of a structured goals of care communication guide. J Palliat Med 2017; 20(9):1004–12.
21. Bernacki RE, Block SD. Communication about serious illness care goals: a review and synthesis of best practices. JAMA Intern Med 2014;174(12):1994–2003.
22. Geerse OP, Lamas DJ, Sanders JJ, et al. A qualitative study of serious illness conversations in patients with advanced cancer. J Palliat Med 2019;1–9. https://doi.org/10.1089/jpm.2018.0487.
23. Schellinger SE, Anderson EW, Frazer MS, et al. Patient self-defined goals: essentials of person-centered care for serious illness. Am J Hosp Palliat Care 2018; 35(1):159–65.
24. Richards CA, Starks H, O'Connor MR, et al. Physicians perceptions of shared decision-making in neonatal and pediatric critical care. Am J Hosp Palliat Care 2018;34(5):669–76.
25. White DB, Malvar G, Karr J, et al. Expanding the paradigm of the physician's role in surrogate decision-making: an empirically derived framework. Crit Care Med 2010;38(3):743–50.
26. Haynes AB, Edmondson L, Lipsitz SR. Mortality trends after a voluntary checklist-based surgical safety collaborative. Ann Surg 2017;266(6):923–9.
27. Mockus Parks S, Winter L, Santana AJ, et al. Family factors in end-of-life decision-making: family conflict and proxy relationships. J Palliat Med 2011;14(2):179–84.
28. Kramer BJ, Kavanaugh M, Trentham-Dietz A, et al. Predictors of family conflict at end of life: the experiences of spouses and adult children of persons with lung cancer. Gerontologist 2009;50(2):215–25.
29. Boelk A, Kramer BJ. Advancing the theory of family conflict at end of life: a hospice case study. J Pain Symptom Manage 2012;44(5):655–69.
30. Vernooij-Dassen M, Draskovic I, McCleery J, et al. Cognitive reframing for cares and people with dementia. Cochrane Database Syst Rev 2011;(11):CD005318.
31. Dolan JG, Veazie PJ. Balance sheets versus decision making dashboards to support treatment choices: a comparative analysis. Patient 2015;8(6):499–505.
32. Akashi A. Ten tips for veterinarians dealing with terminally ill patients. Vet Clin North Am Small Anim Pract 2011;41(3):647–9.
33. Guidelines for critical incidence stress management. American Association of Nurse Anesthetists; 2014. Available at: https://www.aana.com/docs/default-source/practice-aana-com-web-documents-(all)/guidelines-for-critical-incident-stress-management.pdf. Accessed October 31, 2019.
34. Christodoulou-Fella M, Middleton N, Papanthanassoglou EDE, et al. Exploration of the association between nurses' moral distress and secondary traumatic stress syndrome: implications for patient safety in mental health services. Biomed Res Int 2017. https://doi.org/10.1155/2017/1908712.

A Comparison of Human and Animal Assisted Dying Protocols

Beth Marchitelli, DVM, MS[a],*, Jessica Pierce, PhD[b]

KEYWORDS

- Medical aid in dying • Veterinary/human euthanasia • Medical terminology

KEY POINTS

- Verbiage ascribed to the practices of euthanasia for both veterinary and human patients has ethical implications.
- Technical aspects of veterinary and human euthanasia have key similarities and differences.
- Discussion of veterinary and human euthanasia practices has useful insights for both the fields of veterinary medicine and human medicine.

INTRODUCTION

Literature contrasting medical terminology used to describe the ending of life for human patients and for veterinary patients by way of euthanasia is virtually absent from contemporary discussions. Clinical literature comparing the technical aspects of both human euthanasia and veterinary euthanasia also historically has been limited. Although a small number of studies do exist in the human literature[1-5] and veterinary literature independently,[6-15] a direct comparison between human and veterinary euthanasia medical practices and procedures does not. This review places human euthanasia and animal euthanasia side by side, to explore the relevant similarities and differences in the practice of euthanasia between these related fields of medicine, with special focus on the use of medical terminology and technical application of drug protocols. Comparative research in this area may provide useful insights for the fields of veterinary medicine and human medicine alike. This article's central focus is on United States practices; international comparisons are used to highlight important points.

[a] 4 Paws Farewell: Mobile Pet Hospice, Palliative Care and Home Euthanasia, Asheville, NC, USA; [b] Center for Bioethics and Humanities, University of Colorado Anschutz Medical School, Aurora, CO, USA
* Corresponding author.
E-mail address: bmarchitelli@hotmail.com

Vet Clin Small Anim 50 (2020) 617–626
https://doi.org/10.1016/j.cvsm.2019.12.010
0195-5616/20/© 2019 Elsevier Inc. All rights reserved.

MEDICAL TERMINOLOGY
Human Medicine

Terminology relating to human aid in dying (AID) is constantly in flux and without international consensus. In the United States there is little consistency in language, and professional organizations use a range of terms to describe the act of helping medical patients hasten the end of their lives (**Table 1**). For example, the term, *medical AID* (*MAID*), was adopted in 2017 by the American Society of Health-System Pharmacists (HSHP)[16] and is included in their position statement, Pharmacist Participation in Medical Aid in Dying.[17] The term, *physician-assisted dying (PAD)*, is used by the American Academy of Hospice and Palliative Medicine (AAHPM) in their 2016 Statement on Physician-Assisted Dying.[18] The term *physician aid in dying* (PAID) is used by the American Student Medical Association (ASMA) in their bylaws, last amended in 2019.[19] The organization Compassion & Choices uses both AID and MAID on their Web site. In contrast, the older term, *physician-assisted suicide* (*PAS*), used by the American Medical Association (AMA),[20] is currently viewed by most organizations as obsolete and pejorative.

Urging the AMA to follow suit, the American Academy of Family Practitioners (AAFP) broke with the AMA in October of 2018, rejecting their verbiage (PAS) and stance (opposed) in favor of the more progressive terminology (MAID) and position (engaged neutrality).[21]

According to Buchbinder22 in "Choreographing Death: A Social Phenomenology of Medical Aid-in-dying in the United States," "U.S. advocates have recently shifted from PAD (physician aid in dying) to AID (aid in dying)," emphasizing the fact as prescribers, physicians "may play a superficial role in assisted deaths."[22] If the United States finds itself legalizing assisted death by intravenous (IV) injection employed by a physician, this assumption may be challenged.

The term, PAS, has lost favor in the United States due to negative connotations associated with the term, *suicide*. The word, suicide, has been denounced, for instance, by several professional organizations, including HSHP, AAHPM, and AMSA. Nevertheless, the term, *assisted suicide*, is not universally condemned and has some proponents, such as the United States legal and political philosopher Gerald Dworkin and colleagues.[23] The AMA is one of the few professional organizations retaining this now less-favored terminology. The AMA use of PAS, instead of the more progressive terminology, MAID, PAD, PAID, or AID, may reflect their ongoing opposition as an organization to PAD.

In the United States, the only legal form of assisted dying is by medication prescribed by a physician, which the patient must ingest. The terminology (MAID, AID, and PAID) is restricted to describing this process whereby medication is taken orally.

Table 1 Nomenclature used by organizations in the United States	
American Society of Health-System Pharmacists	Medical aid in dying (MAID)
American Association of Hospice and Palliative Medicine	Physician-assisted dying (PAD)
American Medical Student Association	Physician aid in dying (PAID)
American Association of Family Practitioners	Medical aid in dying (MAID)
Compassion & Choices	Aid in dying (AID); medical aid in dying (MAID)
American Medical Association	Physician-assisted suicide (PAS)

In contrast, medically assisted death in Canada, the Netherlands, Belgium, Luxembourg, and Columbia is permitted by both the patient self-administered oral route and by medication given IV by a physician.

Professional medical organizations in the United States universally avoid the term, *euthanasia*. Compassion & Choices, for example, rejects the term, euthanasia, because "in the act of euthanasia, the physician—not the dying person—chooses and acts to cause the death of the patient."[24] By comparison, when the term, euthanasia, is used in the Netherlands in the context of MAID, it functions to distinguish the route of administration of life-ending medication (IV, as opposed to oral) and does not reflect who is responsible for making the decision to end life, which is presumably always the patient. In the Netherlands, euthanasia refers to the facilitation of death by a physician administering life-ending medication IV; PAS refers to life-ending medication prescribed by a physician and taken orally by the patient. This distinction is captured in the Dutch guidelines for physicians and pharmacists entitled, "KNMG/KNMP Guidelines for the Practice of Euthanasia and Physician-Assisted Suicide" (August 2012).[25]

The Dutch word for PAS, used in the guidelines referenced previously, is *hulp bij zelfdoding*. This phrase literally means "help with suicide."[26] The Dutch language offers considerable nuance: the word, *zelfdoding*, was chosen over the word, *zelfmoord*, which translates as "self-murder." The latter carries a negative connotation and implies that one has taken one's own life under duress, which more closely resembles the English interpretation of the word, suicide.

The term, *death with dignity*, generally is associated with legal statutes, as seen, for example, in the name of the acts legalizing MAID in Oregon and Washington. The nomenclature of legal statutes also varies widely, as reflected in **Table 2**.

Ongoing public and professional discourse surrounding appropriate ascription of terms to life-ending acts in human medicine highlights one of the most striking differences between the human and veterinary medical fields. Where human medicine has inadvertently complicated discourse through the use of multiple terms, veterinary medicine has overly simplified discussion through lack of a nuanced vocabulary.

Veterinary Medicine

In contrast to human medicine, veterinary medicine has an extremely simple—and, it might be argued, simplistic—vocabulary for talking about interventions that hasten or bring about death. The single term, euthanasia, is used to describe the vast ethical and moral landscape of ending the lives of animals in a variety of settings.

The American Veterinary Medical Association (AVMA) uses the term, euthanasia, to refer to a broad range of both techniques and motivations for deliberately ending the

Table 2 Language used in United States legislation	
Oregon	Oregon Death with Dignity Act, 1994/1997
Washington	Washington Death with Dignity Act, 2008
Vermont	Patient Choice and Control at the End of Life Act, 2013
California	End of Life Option Act, 2015/2016
Colorado	End of Life Options Act, 2016
District of Columbia	D.C. Death with Dignity Act, 2016/2017
Hawaii	Our Care, Our Choice Act, 2018/2019

Data from Death with dignity: current death with dignity laws. Available at: https://www.deathwithdignity.org/learn/death-with-dignity-acts/. Accessed January 12, 2019.

lives of animals. Euthanasia broadly covers any killing that is "humanely" executed and that relieves suffering, whether this suffering is natural (eg, the result of illness) or directly inflicted by human activities (eg, in a laboratory research setting). The 2013 edition of the AVMA Guidelines for the Euthanasia of Animals describes "humane technique" vaguely as death that is taken with "the highest degree of respect, and with an emphasis on making the death as painless and distress free as possible."[27]

The AVMA acknowledges the moral complexity of killing practices and the potential ethical complications of using the same terminology to describe the compassionate hastening of death for an extremely ill companion animal and to the killing of laboratory animals or healthy animals in an overcrowded shelter. Nonetheless, the AVMA guidelines do not attempt to nuance the language of animal death. Although the guidelines advise against euthanasia in some situations, such as the so-called convenience euthanasia of a healthy dog or cat at the request of the owner, they nevertheless fail to provide an alternative term for this form of killing.

Sidestepping the most serious potential terminological issues with euthanasia, the AVMA uses separate language to describe the killing of food animals and the mass killing of agricultural animals affected by natural disaster or disease by creating separate documents for these forms of killing. These guidelines use the words, *slaughter*[28] and *depopulation*,[29–31] in their titles to address the obvious practical and moral differences in killing practices.

Colloquially and most commonly, euthanasia is used to describe the ending of the lives of companion animals suffering from debilitating life-limiting illness. The terminology, AID or assisted death, is never used by the AVMA, perhaps because the veterinary profession does not routinely assign agency to animals, and animals are not given a voice in the decision to die. Even in cases where hospice care has been instituted and where terminology, such as *hastening death* or *assisted dying*, might be appropriate, the language of euthanasia is still the profession's term of art. Veterinarians working in companion animal care thus often resort to euphemisms and soft metaphors, such as "helping" animals, "giving an animal her wings," or giving the "gift" of hastened death. If any nuance is to be found, it is in the occasional use of the term, *natural death*, to distinguish deaths that have occurred without the direct intervention of a veterinary professional. The term, natural death, has created some concerns within the veterinary profession because of the appeal of the concept of naturalness and the fear that in seeking a natural death for their companion, pet owners will allow animals to die without adequate (or any) supportive palliative care.

EUTHANASIA PROTOCOLS

This section gives a brief overview of the legal and historical landscape of human and animal euthanasia protocols, to provide context for the primary focus, which is the actual medical/pharmaceutical tools used to induce death in human euthanasia compared with animal euthanasia. The term, euthanasia, is used to refer to life-ending medication given IV; PAD, to refer to life-ending medication ingested orally; and MAID, as an umbrella term encompassing both. Examination of human oral drug protocols for PAD is omitted, because the IV route is more readily comparable to animal euthanasia practices. Regardless, oral drug protocols for human euthanasia are pertinent to the discussion at large, specifically in light of the variety of drug protocols used in the United States for this purpose. Given the physiologic similarities, it might be assumed the path to achieving a painless and quick death would be similar, but human euthanasia and PAID protocols differ from animal protocols in several ways. The reasons why veterinarians use certain drugs whereas physicians use others are complex, related to historical development of euthanasia rather than to physiologic differences in how painless and quick death can best be achieved. An overview of this extraordinarily complex terrain is provided. This is an area in need of considerably more research and discussion.

There have been progressive developments in both human euthanasia/PAD and animal euthanasia protocols around the world over the past several decades. This landscape is dynamic and evolving, and what is presented in this article is a snapshot of this moment in time. PAD has been practiced in Switzerland since as early as the 1940s. PAD has been legal in Finland since 2012 and Germany since 2015. The Netherlands was one of the first countries to legalize human euthanasia and PAD in 2002. Belgium also legalized human euthanasia in 2002 and became the first country to legalize human euthanasia for minors in 2014. Other countries where human euthanasia is legal include Luxembourg (legalized in 2009), Columbia (legalized in 2015), and Canada (legalized in 2016). In the United States, PAD is legal in 6 states—Oregon, Washington, Vermont, Colorado, California, and Hawaii—and in the District of Columbia. Human euthanasia is illegal in all 50 US states.

In the United States and elsewhere, the reaction from the human medical community to involvement in MAID has spanned from willing participation to reluctance and refusal. Some physicians contend that participation in MAID directly violates the physician's Hippocratic Oath. Physician groups also have refused to carry out capital punishment by lethal injection, arguing that it violates the commitment to "do no harm." In contrast to the physician's oath, which offers physicians an ethical way out of participation in MAID, the veterinary oath endorses and even promotes the act of euthanasia as "the prevention and relief of animal suffering."[32]

The AVMA had actively worked to remain outside the debate surrounding human euthanasia and assisted dying as well as outside the conversation about lethal injection in capital punishment. Mainly, the AVMA has distanced itself by simply not talking about human euthanasia at all. But in a singular exception to this rule of silence, Gail Golab, director of the AVMA Animal Welfare Division from 2007 to 2015, elucidated the scope of the AVMA guidelines on euthanasia. The guidelines, she wrote, "were developed to provide guidance for veterinarians when euthanizing animals. They are not intended to serve as guidelines for the euthanasia of human beings."[33]

Human Euthanasia Protocols

Human euthanasia has been legal in the Netherlands since 2002. In the 15 years since legalization, Dutch physicians and pharmacists have been working to refine drug protocols for human euthanasia. The Dutch experience thus provides the most extensive effort to develop effective drug protocols for human euthanasia. The Royal Dutch Association for the Advancement of Pharmacy (KNMP) and Royal Dutch Medical Association (KNMG) joint guidelines stipulate a 2-part process. A medical coma is first induced, followed by the administration of a neuromuscular blocking agent[25] (**Table 3**). The administration of the benzodiazepine midazolam prior to coma induction is permissible if the patient would like a reduction in consciousness during the transition from the waking state to coma.

Table 3 Royal Dutch Association for the Advancement of Pharmacy/Royal Dutch Medical Association guidelines for the practice of euthanasia	
Part 1	Coma induction: sodium thiopental, 2000 mg/propofol, 1000 mg IV
Part 2	Neuromuscular blocking agent: rocuronium, 150 mg IV

Part one: medical coma induction
A standard dose of 2000 mg of sodium thiopental or 1000 mg of propofol has been established to reduce medication dosing errors.[25] One of these 2 coma-inducing medications is to be given IV in less than 5 minutes directly by a physician or via the elastomeric infusion pump to achieve a medically induced coma. The elastomeric pump is a mechanical pump, which the patient can control and can use to self-administer IV medication. Once the physician is confident that a medically induced coma has been achieved, a neuromuscular blocking agent is administered. The importance of verifying that a medically induced coma has been achieved prior to administration of the neuromuscular blocking agent is emphasized in the KNMP/KNMG guidelines.[25]

Part two: neuromuscular blocking agent
In the Netherlands, the most common neuromuscular blocking agent used is rocuronium. The use of a neuromuscular blocking agent is mandated regardless of whether death has occurred from the coma-inducing medication. Neuromuscular blocking agents are included in the protocol based on historical precedent and to mitigate adverse events that might occur with administration of high doses of sodium or propofol alone. For some patients, clinical death does occur before administration of the neuromuscular blocking agent.

In a study from 2000, in the Netherlands, the incidence of complications was 7% for PAD and 3% for euthanasia. Complications included such things as "myoclonus, nausea and vomiting." Problems with completion occurred 16% of the time for PAD and 6% for euthanasia.[1] Several other studies have evaluated technical problems and preferences in the technical application of MAID in the Netherlands.[2–5] Some of these studies evaluate data collected prior to the official codification of such practices into Dutch law. Contemporary complication rates of euthanasia in the Netherlands may be significantly reduced, as a result of legalization in 2002 and the standardization of drug protocols. At present, complication data from other countries where human euthanasia is legal are minimal.[34]

Animal Euthanasia Protocols

Sodium pentobarbital products are the primary means by which companion animal euthanasia is achieved. Sodium pentobarbital combination products are approved for euthanasia in dogs, cats, and large animals by the Center for Veterinary Medicine (CVM), the arm of the Food and Drug Administration (FDA) responsible for veterinary drug approval. Dosages for products containing sodium pentobarbital and phenytoin are labeled as 1 mL per 4.5 kg of body weight for dogs.[34] Single-agent sodium pentobarbital products are recognized by the CVM/FDA and also are labeled for use in dogs, horses, small mammals, and rodents.[35] In clinical practice, the dose delivered of pentobarbital products may far exceed the labeled dose.[7]

Practices vary considerably on the use of sedating medication prior to administration of sodium pentobarbital products, to reduce fear and anxiety for both the pet and pet owner and to help alleviate adverse events during and after the euthanasia process. Sedation protocols prior to euthanasia commonly include opioids and sedatives in the form of phenothiazines, α_2-agonists, dissociative drugs, and benzodiazepines (**Table 4**). A small number of studies do exist comparing various sedation protocols prior to the administration of euthanasia solution.[6–8]

There are few studies in the veterinary literature that quantify adverse events or side effects during the euthanasia process that may be disturbing to animals or to humans performing or witnessing the procedure. These side effects include agonal respiration, vomiting, tremors, vocalization, and technical problems with completion.[6–15] These

| Table 4 |
| Drugs commonly used for the euthanasia of companion animals |

Part 1: Presedation	Phenothiazines, α_2-agonists, opioids, dissociative drugs, benzodiazepines, hypnotic agents (propofol)
Part 2	Sodium pentobarbital/sodium Pentobarbital + phenytoin sodium IV

studies are outdated and do not include commonly used sedation protocols or euthanasia solutions currently on the market.

The AVMA guidelines on euthanasia include substantial detail regarding appropriate and inappropriate methods of achieving humane euthanasia in a wide range of animal species (excluding, of course, the human animal).[27] Specifically, neuromuscular blocking agents are considered unacceptable as a sole method of euthanasia and should not be given in the same syringe as a sodium pentobarbital product. The specific guidelines regarding neuromuscular blocking agents are in place to help avoid inappropriate administration of these agents. In particular, neuromuscular blocking agents should not be used without the appropriate absence of consciousness, because of the potential for animal suffering. For example, the euthanasia solution T-61 was voluntarily removed from the market in the United States in 1989 because of the inclusion of the neuromuscular blocker mebezonium.[36] Assurance that animals would be incontrovertibly unconscious prior to the effects of mebezonium could not be proved,[12–14] despite efforts to do so.[10] In the United States, Georgia has made the administration of neuromuscular blocking agents in lieu of sodium pentobarbital products illegal for the euthanasia of dogs and cats.[37–40] Many other state laws forbid the application of neuromuscular blocking agents as sole agents of euthanasia. Veterinary medicine's experience over many decades with sodium pentobarbital alone or in combination with phenytoin has proved that, for animals, a humane, peaceful, and successful death can be achieved without the administration of a neuromuscular blocking agent. The addition of sedative medication prior to euthanasia may more reliably assure death that is achieved in such a way as to minimize adverse events for pets and family members. To date, there are no studies supporting or refuting this point despite a substantial amount of anecdotal evidence. Direct extrapolation to human medical protocols should be approached critically and with caution. Although dogs and cats are similar to humans, there also are profound differences that could be relevant to this discussion.

USE OF NEUROMUSCULAR BLOCKING AGENTS IN LETHAL INJECTION IN RELATIONSHIP TO HUMAN AND ANIMAL EUTHANASIA PROTOCOLS

It is difficult to have a discussion about human and animal euthanasia protocols without mentioning the controversy surrounding the inclusion of neuromuscular blocking agents in protocols of lethal injection in the United States. (Lethal injection is illegal in most European countries, so the debates over lethal injection and assisted death more easily remain separated.) Inexperienced and untrained staff and restricted access to specific medications have led to the highly publicized deaths of several inmates in the United States, who unquestionably experienced unnecessary suffering. Controversy primarily arises in relation to the inclusion of neuromuscular blocking medication, which is not included in veterinary euthanasia protocols but is part of human euthanasia protocols in the Netherlands and Canada.

The inclusion of neuromuscular blocking medication in human euthanasia protocols as the standard of care is not discussed in the argument against their use in lethal injection. Successful and humane administration of neuromuscular blocking agents as part of a euthanasia drug protocol is inextricably linked to the expertise of the professional administering the medication. Experienced practitioners in the Netherlands have included such agents for a variety of reasons, including the mitigation of side effects that may be unpleasant for family members, assurance of completion of the death process, and the avoidance of side effects when administering coma-inducing agents alone. The human medical field is also very familiar with using neuromuscular blocking agents for routine surgical procedures. Neuromuscular blocking agents are used to facilitate intubation and in cases of thoracic or abdominal surgery. Veterinary medicine does not use such agents for routine surgical procedures. Neuromuscular blocking agents are not present in most veterinary hospitals, aside from large referral centers and universities. As discussed previously, many states in the United States have statutes against the use of neuromuscular blocking agents for the euthanasia of animals. The legal status of neuromuscular blocking agents in the euthanasia of animals, their inclusion in some lethal injection protocols, and the legitimacy of neuromuscular blocking agents in human euthanasia protocols in the Netherlands add much confusion in drawing comparisons between human and animal protocols.

SUMMARY

Comparative research in the use of terminology and drug protocols for human and animal euthanasia may provide useful insights for the fields of veterinary and human medicine alike. In addition to medical and legal comparisons, there is rich potential in a comparison of the ethical decision-making matrices that shape terminology and techniques in the practice of human versus veterinary euthanasia.

DISCLOSURE

The authors have nothing to disclose.

REFERENCES

1. Groenewoud JH, Van der Heide A, Onwuteaka-Philipsen BD, et al. Clinical problems with the performance of euthanasia and physician-assisted suicide in the Netherlands. N Engl J Med 2000;342(8):551–6.
2. Sprij B. Could it be a little less? Let the dose of thiopental in euthanasia depend on body weight. Ned Tijdschr Geneeskd 2010;154:A1983.
3. Horikx A, Admiraal PV. Utilization of euthanatic agents; experience of physicians with 227 patients, 1998 – 2000. Ned Tijdschr Geneeskd 2000;144:2497–500.
4. Lalmohamed A, Horikx A. Experience with euthanasia since 2007. Analysis of problems with execution. Ned Tijdschr Geneeskd 2010;154:A1882.
5. Kouwenhoven PSC, van Thiel GJMW, Raijmakers NJH, et al. Euthanasia or physician-assisted suicide? A survey from the Netherlands. Eur J Gen Pract 2014;20:25–31.
6. Ramsay EC, Wetzel RW. Comparison of five regimes for oral administration of medication to induce sedation in dogs prior to euthanasia. J Am Vet Med Assoc 1998;213(2):240–2.
7. Wetzel RW, Ramsay EC. Comparison of four regimes for intraoral administration of medication to induce sedation in cats prior to euthanasia. J Am Vet Med Assoc 1998;213(2):243–5.

8. Bullock J, Lanaux T, Buckley G. Comparison of euthanasia methods 343 client-owned dogs: pentobarbital/phenytoin alone vs propofol and pentobarbital/phenytoin combination. Abstract IVECCS Conference. 2016. Available at: http://2016.iveccs.org/twocol.aspx?page=Small+Animal+Abstract. Accessed January 12, 2019.

9. Evans AT, Broadstone R, Stapleton J, et al. Comparison of pentobarbital alone and pentobarbital in combination with lidocaine for euthanasia in dogs. J Am Vet Med Assoc 1993;203(5):664–6.

10. Hellebrekers LJ, Baumans V, Bertens AP, et al. On the use of T61 for euthanasia of domestic and laboratory animals; an ethical evaluation. Lab Anim 1990;24:200–4.

11. Wallach MB, Peterson KE, Richards RK. Electrophysiologic studies of a combination of secobarbital and dibucaine for euthanasia of dogs. Am J Vet Res 1981; 42(5):850–3.

12. Lumb WV, Doshi J, Scott RJ. A comparative study of T-61 pentobarbital for euthanasia of dogs. J Am Vet Med Assoc 1978;172(2):149–52.

13. Rowan AN. T-61 use in the euthanasia of domestic animals: a survey. In: Fox MW, Mickley LD, editors. Advances in animal welfare science. Washington, DC: Humane Society of the US; 1985. p. 79–86.

14. Barocio LD. Review of literature on use of T-61 as an euthanasic agent. Int J Study Anim Probl 1983;4(4):336–42.

15. Chalifoux A, Dallaire A. Physiologic and behavioral evaluation of CO euthanasia of adult dogs. Am J Vet Res 1983;44(12):2412–7.

16. Cobaugh DJ. Medical aid in dying. Am J Health Syst Pharm 2017;74(16):1214–5.

17. American Society of Health-System Pharmacists. Professional policies approved by the 2017 ASHP House of Delegates. Am J Health Syst Pharm 2017;74:e430–4.

18. American Academy of Hospice and Palliative Medicine position Statement. 2016. Available at: http://aahpm.org/positions/pad. Accessed January 12, 2019

19. American Medical Student Association. 2019. Available at: https://www.amsa.org/wp-content/uploads/2019/05/2019_CBIA.pdf. Accessed January 27, 2020.

20. American Medical Association Physician-Assisted Suicide Code of Medical Ethics Opinion. 5.7. Copyright 1995-2019. Available at: https://www.ama-assn.org/delivering-care/ethics/physician-assisted-suicide. Accessed January 12, 2019.

21. Grube D. American Academy of family physicians adopts new position of "engaged neutrality" on medical aid in dying. 2018. Available at: https://compassionandchoices.org/news/american-academy-family-physicians-adopts-new-position-engaged-neutrality-medical-aid-dying/. Accessed February 21, 2019.

22. Buchbinder M. Choreographing death: a social phenomenology of medical aid-in-dying in the United States. Med Anthropol Q 2018;32(4):481–97.

23. Dworkin G, Frey RG, Bok S. Euthanasia and physician-assisted suicide. Cambridge: Cambridge University Press; 1998.

24. Compassion and choices. Glossary of terms. 2019. Available at: https://compassionandchoices.org/end-of-life-planning/learn/glossary-of-terms/. Accessed January 12, 2019.

25. KNMG/KNMP guidelines for the practice of euthanasia and physician-assisted suicide. Available at: https://www.knmp.nl/downloads/guidelines-for-the-practice-of-euthanasia.pdf. Accessed January 12, 2019.

26. ten Have H, Welie J. Death and medical power: an ethical analysis of dutch euthanasia practice. New York: Open University Press; 2005. p. 211.

27. AVMA guidelines for the euthanasia of animals: 2013 edition. Available at: https://www.avma.org/KB/Policies/Documents/euthanasia.pdf. Accessed January 12, 2019.

28. AVMA guidelines for the humane slaughter of animals: 2016 edition. 2016. Available at: https://www.avma.org/KB/Resources/Reference/AnimalWelfare/Documents/Humane-Slaughter-Guidelines.pdf. Accessed January 12, 2019.

29. AVMA guidance on emergency animal depopulation. 2018. Available at: https://www.avma.org/News/JAVMANews/Pages/180601b.aspx. Accessed January 12, 2019.

30. Dyer O, White C, García Rada A. Assisted dying: law and practice around the world. BMJ 2015;351:h4481.

31. Muller MD. Attention to language in a request for physician aid in dying. Am J Hosp Palliat Care 2011;28(1):63–4.

32. American Veterinary Medical Association. Veterinarian's oath. 2019. Available at: https://www.avma.org/News/JAVMANews/Pages/071215a.aspx. Accessed January 12, 2019.

33. Nolan S. Lethal injection opponents use AVMA euthanasia guidelines to make their case. 2007. Available at: https://www.avma.org/News/JAVMANews/Pages/071215a.aspx. Accessed January 12, 2019.

34. Deirick S. Euthanasia practice in Belgium : a population-based evaluation of trends and currently debated issues. 2018. Available at: https://www.worldrtd.net/sites/default/files/newsfiles/Sigrid_Dierickx.pdf. Accessed January 27, 2020.

35. Plumb's veterinary drug handbook. 2017. Available at: https://www.plumbsveterinarydrugs.com/#!/monograph/cpicfuyBJo/. Accessed January 12, 2019.

36. National Research Council (US). Committee on pain and distress in laboratory animals. Recognition and alleviation of pain and distress in laboratory animals. Washington (DC): National Academies Press (US); 1992. Chapter 7: Euthanasia. Available at: https://www.ncbi.nlm.nih.gov/books/NBK235440/.

37. Alper T. Anesthetizing the public conscience: lethal injection and animal euthanasia, 35 Fordham Urb. L.J. 817. 2008. Available at: https://scholarship.law.berkeley.edu/facpubs/835/. Accessed January 12, 2019.

38. Eyre-Pugh RE, Yeates JW. Treatment, palliative care or euthanasia? Comparing end of life issues in veterinary and human medicine. Preprints 2017. https://doi.org/10.20944/preprints201708.0094.v1.

39. Meijer EVA. The good life, the good death: companion animals and euthanasia. Anim Stud J 2018;7(1):20–225.

40. van Herten J. Killing of companion animals: to be avoided at all costs?. In: Meijboom LB, Stassen EN, editors. The end of animal life: a start for ethical debate. Wageningen, The Netherlands: Wageningen Academic Publishers; 2016. p. 203–23. https://doi.org/10.3920/978-90-8686-808-7_13.

Nonpharmacologic Methods to Improve the Euthanasia Experience

Tamara Shearer, DVM, MS

KEYWORDS

- Euthanasia • Death and dying • Animal hospice • Aid in dying • Euthanasia support

KEY POINTS

- Implementation of a hospice care plan can help support veterinary patients and their owners and improve the euthanasia experience.
- Evaluation of the pet owner's psychosocial needs provides benefits for the patient, the pet owner, and the veterinarian by improving the efficiency of care.
- Environmental enrichment to improve the atmosphere of a veterinary practice improves the euthanasia experience.
- Mindful scheduling of elective euthanasia procedures during quiet hospital times may be less stressful for the pet owner, staff, and veterinarian.

INTRODUCTION

In addition to the careful selection of drug choice, route of delivery, and rate of delivery of euthanasia drugs, veterinarians have a responsibility to provide a good death by implementing nonpharmacologic methods to support the client and patient surrounding the euthanasia process. Often simple, commonsense methods and approaches can help to minimize the stress surrounding euthanasia and provide a better experience for the patient and client. This may also benefit the veterinarian and staff by making the procedure a more organized event with less pressure, tension, and worry.

It is preferred and hoped that animal patients have been enrolled in a hospice and palliative care plan before the decision to euthanize. Research studies have documented that human patients enrolled in a hospice care plan have a longer, better quality of life and their family members have a shorter grieving period.[1] Because of the bond between people and their pets, similar benefits likely apply to veterinary medicine.

Unfortunately, not all clients are able to benefit from hospice and palliative care for their pets or it may not be possible with patients that succumb to an acute crises. The

Smoky Mountain Integrative Veterinary Clinic, 1054 Haywood Road Suite 3, Sylva, NC 28779, USA
E-mail address: tshearer5@frontier.com

Vet Clin Small Anim 50 (2020) 627–638
https://doi.org/10.1016/j.cvsm.2019.12.011
0195-5616/20/© 2020 Elsevier Inc. All rights reserved.

Box 1
Five-step strategy for comprehensive palliative and hospice care

Step 1: Evaluation of the pet owner's needs, beliefs, and goals for the pet (psychosocial needs)

Step 2: Education about the disease process or euthanasia process

Step 3: Development of a personalized plan for the pet and pet owner

Step 4: Application of palliative or hospice care techniques

Step 5: Emotional support during hospice care process and after the death of the pet

---

following material introduces how applying the philosophy of hospice care can improve the euthanasia experience and includes practical tips for patients not enrolled in a hospice care plan.

HOSPICE CARE AND PALLIATIVE TO IMPROVE THE EUTHANASIA EXPERIENCE

An integrative hospice care plan is supportive of all aspects surrounding death including the euthanasia process. Use of the five-step Hospice and Palliative Care Plan provides guidelines that include a template to include nonpharmacologic support that covers comfort care surrounding time of death. Developed in 2006, this protocol serves as a template to organize animal hospice and palliative care so that no part of support for patient or family is overlooked (**Box 1**).[2,3] A modification of that plan has been created specifically for euthanasia to improve the experience for the pet owner, veterinarian, and staff (**Box 2**).

Step 1: Evaluation of the Pet Owner's Needs, Beliefs, and Preferences Regarding Euthanasia (Psychosocial Needs)

Evaluation of the pet owner's psychosocial needs, beliefs, and goals for the pet sets the foundation for the best personalized euthanasia experience. A pet owner's needs, beliefs, and goals are shaped by all of life's experiences, positive and negative, and have an effect on how they approach end-of-life choices and euthanasia preferences. Psychosocial needs are evaluated by asking the appropriate questions, including open-ended questions, making observations, and knowing that needs may transform as a condition or situation progresses. It allows the practitioner to understand and define the needs of the pet and pet owner. For example, an individual with a negative euthanasia experience may be in need of more support. Reassurance that the pet will not be separated from the owner may help ease anxiety for an owner that heard their

---
Box 2
Modified five-step strategy for hospice care with euthanasia focus

Step 1: Evaluation of the pet owner's needs, beliefs, and preferences regarding euthanasia (psychosocial needs)

Step 2: Education about the euthanasia process

Step 3: Development of a personalized plan for the euthanasia based on the information gathered in Step 1

Step 4: Organize and carry out the euthanasia

Step 5: Emotional support during the hospice care process and after the death of the pet

---

previous pet cry out when it was separated from them for intravenous catheter placement.

Taking the time to investigate the needs, beliefs, and preferences of the client before euthanasia offers many benefits to the client and veterinary practitioner (**Box 3**). It not only influences how a patient will be treated but also improves the client-patient-doctor relationship through better communication. It helps define what options or techniques are used to support the patient. It also improves the efficiency of care when there are time-sensitive issues, such as the need for an urgent euthanasia because of increased suffering. All of this helps to put the caretaker at ease and also should enhance the trust and respect for the veterinarian's recommendations. This lessens the emotional side effects for the family and may minimize conflict among veterinarian, family, and family members.

An important part of gathering information that helps prepare for a euthanasia should include details about the pet's relationship to the pet owner. An overview of the pet owner's support system of family, friends, and clergy is also helpful in understanding areas of deficiencies so extra resources can be provided or suggested.

Information about the pet's current activities of daily living may also help to shape a tailored plan for the family. This process also helps to determine if modifications need to be made to the patient's environment to prevent injuries or make it easier for the pet to ambulate before euthanasia. It also helps to provide creative ideas for special euthanasia locations. For example, the pet owners may appreciate the option of having their dog euthanized on the shore of a lake if the dog had a passion for swimming. Likewise, a special place for a kitty may be the porch where they liked to lay in the sun.

Taking the time to investigate needs may help the practitioner to understand the pet's acceptance and behavior toward medical care so modifications in procedures can be made. Pet owners should be able to describe how the pet acts when he/she is at a veterinary hospital. Pets that have had a stressful event or experienced anxiety when interacting with members of the veterinary team are best addressed with a fear-free approach. Creative thinking Is useful in minimizing stress. Pets that are fearful or anxious when entering a veterinary hospital may benefit from having a euthanasia house call or if possible an oral anxiolytic drug before travel.

Veterinarians should have a good understanding of the family's beliefs about death and dying when developing a plan for the patient. Before euthanasia, the pet owners should be asked about their beliefs in euthanasia, natural death, and the use of proportionate palliative sedation if symptom management fails to keep their pet

---

Box 3
Benefits of evaluating caretaker's psychosocial needs before euthanasia

Improves client-patient-doctor relationship

Influences how the euthanasia is carried out

Influences the selection of timing of euthanasia

Improves the efficiency of care or euthanasia when there are time-sensitive issues

Strengthens communication

Helps put the caretaker at ease

Enhances trust and respect for veterinarian

Lessens the emotional side effects for the family

Minimizes conflict between veterinarian, family, and family members

comfortable. The pet owner should be prepared ahead of time for the choices available when making final arrangements so they have time to pick the best options for their family and their pet.

If needed, a review of psychosocial needs may be helpful when there is conflict between members of the family or care team surrounding the time of euthanasia. The process of decline as death approaches is ever changing and unpredictable. A pet owner's perspective may transform as the time nears for euthanasia.

The worksheet in **Fig. 1** provides practical guidance to organize critical information during this emotional and stressful time.

Step 2: Education About the Disease and/or Euthanasia Process

Typically, education and the planning for the death and dying process should start early once the pet has a grave prognosis because it is the first step in the preparation for bereavement. A description of the dying process, whether by natural disease progression or by euthanasia intervention, should be shared with the pet owner based on the specific disease trajectory before the death of the pet. Education about the euthanasia process is best carried out by the veterinarian and technical support staff. A veterinarian should be able to share what to expect when the pet is nearing death, and explain the euthanasia and the dying process. Education about the euthanasia process should be based on the pet owner's background, past experiences, and their "need to know." These insights should become clear after the initial evaluation of the client's psychosocial needs and euthanasia preferences. It is important to be sensitive and mindful about how the information is being received and to be capable of modifying or postponing the amount of information shared. A recent article by Borden and colleagues[4] highlighted the importance of the elicitation of the client's perspectives and psychosocial needs in the context of euthanasia discussions, identifying the need for improvement in the area of veterinary communication.

Until it is time for euthanasia, pet owners should be educated on how to recognize the clinical signs of disease because some debilitated patients cannot communicate their need for pain and symptom relief. It is better to proactively treat for symptoms than to undertreat clinical signs to ensure everything is being done to enhance quality of life. At the very least, the pet owner should be taught how to recognize pain, nausea, dehydration, constipation, dyspnea, melena, anemia, seizures, urinary tract infections, and urinary obstructions. Pet owners should be taught to report health changes to prevent suffering so the veterinarian can modify the treatment plan or share the option of euthanasia.

There are specific signs of approaching death that may alert the pet owner that time remaining with their pet is limited. Not all clinical signs of a disease in an individual are the same and not all signs of death are the same. Whether a patient is in hospice care or not, a pet owner should be aware of how to recognize if a pet is actively dying.

A review of the process of euthanasia is important to share with the caretaker based on the veterinarian's euthanasia protocol. The practitioner should share what the pet might experience and what the pet owner will see during the euthanasia process. Pet owners need to be aware that adverse events can occur. The American Veterinary Medical Association Guidelines for the Euthanasia of Animals describes "disturbing" events during the euthanasia process.[5] The guidelines state that the release of inhibition of motor activity may be accompanied by vocalization and muscle contractions during loss of consciousness similar to what is observed during anesthesia. During sedation when the righting reflex has been lost, reflex struggling, vocalization, and convulsions may also occur. They make note in the guidelines that these changes

Caretaker data	Record information below
Primary caretaker	
Description of problem and reasons for euthanasia	
Family members and ages	
Available physical support	
Available emotional support	
Is caretaker responsible for family members with health issues	
If caretaker responsible for young children, what is their relationship to the pet?	
Schedule flexibility (retired, full time, part time, works at home?)	
Worries about cost of care?	
Environment and activities of daily living	
Patient's past lifestyle (working dog, agility, companion)	
Pet's activities of daily living (mobility capability, grooming habits…)	
Floor type	
Steps	
Outside terrain	
Explore pet's behavior	
Current behavior at home with family members	
Current behavior at home with other animals	
Behavior outside of home with new people	
Behavior outside the home with animals	
Tolerance or behavior in a hospital setting	
Preference for warmth versus cool	
Past Medical Experiences	
Positive experiences	
Negative experiences	
Losses	
Details of the past that need to be avoided	
Past trouble caring for the patient	
Philosophy on death and end-of-life choices	
Belief regarding natural death	
Belief regarding hospice assisted death	
Belief on euthanasia	
Preference to where pet dies	
Pet owners desire to be present	
Choice on how to handle the remains	

Fig. 1. Psychosocial needs: euthanasia worksheet.

"may be disturbing to observers," which is one of the reasons it is important to educate clients on these changes.

Most conversations with the pet owner should include discussions about the administration of drugs and the physical changes that may occur during the sedation and euthanasia process. Some adverse events during the euthanasia process include agitation, myoclonus, twitching or tremors, vocalization, agonal respirations, Cheyne-Stokes respirations or irregular breathing patterns, opisthotonic posturing, and release of urine and feces. These responses to the sedatives and euthanasia solutions plus natural reflexes can be distressful to witness even by the most informed client and seasoned veterinarian. Preparing the client for potential adverse events witnessed during the euthanasia process can offset unnecessary distress. However, even the most well prepared client finds some events haunting. A small group of clients that were educated about the clinical changes surrounding death were polled at this author's clinic (Smoky Mountain Integrative Veterinary Clinic) and reported that one of the most distressing adverse events witnessed was when their pet experienced agonal respirations.

Many practitioners have developed a special dialogue to communicate the details of euthanasia. A sample dialogue that is often used by this author to describe the euthanasia process is found in **Box 4**.

Step 3: Development of a Personalized Plan for the Euthanasia

The development of a personalized plan for the euthanasia should take into consideration the psychosocial beliefs of the family and their desires for the pet. The veterinarian's prime responsibility is to set up a plan that works for the pet and family. This includes organizing a care team that meets the emotional needs of the pet owner. It is also important to treat all processes that interfere with quality of life until the time for euthanasia. Even in the last days, a veterinarian should attempt to treat conditions that cause distress, such as severe otitis externa or keratoconjunctivitis sicca. Next are guidelines to help structure a personalized care plan.

Make 24-hour care available

The first step for peace of mind for the caretaker is to make sure the pet owner knows how to get help anytime the animal is in a crisis. A team approach using other

---

Box 4
Sample euthanasia dialog: veterinarian to client

"When I euthanize a pet it is a peaceful process. I start with a sedative injection that goes under the skin with a tiny needle. That injection relaxes the pet and makes the patient unconscious. They might be feeling the best that they have felt in some time because they will become unaware of any distress and it will make any pain dissipate. The sedation shot that transitions them to become unconscious takes about 10 to 20 minutes to work.

Once the pet is unconscious, I give the euthanasia solution which is pentobarbital and it will function like an anesthetic overdose shutting down the pet's systems. The passing is typically very peaceful. There may be natural reflexes during the process that might occur that pet is unaware of but may be difficult for pet owners to witness. Not all pets exhibit those reflexes but they include breathing fast and irregular, there can be twitching, and deep or agonal breaths with their mouth opening wide, they may also urinate or defecate. It is also natural for the pet's eyes to remain open even after death. Not often but some pets will vocalize sometime during the process. I have to emphasize that these observations, if they do occur, are reflexes and are natural phenomenon. A pet is not aware that these things are happening. Again my goal is to make this process as peaceful as possible. Do you have any questions about what I just discussed?"

professionals plays an important role in providing 24-hour care so the entire burden of urgent care does not fall on one individual, who in the past was usually the primary veterinarian. Some practitioners provide a crisis kit containing various medications and aids to help manage any clinical signs until a veterinarian is reached. To provide comprehensive care, the hospice care team should incorporate a pet loss support hotline and emergency clinic contact information for the pet owner.

Provide the proper hospital environment for euthanasia

A practice that specializes in hospice and palliative care may have already created an environment conducive to being peaceful and fear-free. Some busy general practices may find this to be a challenge. Environmental enrichment can greatly enhance the euthanasia experience. Providing nonslip flooring for dogs that can still ambulate is important to prevent falls. Routine examination rooms can be transformed into a comfortable space by replacing fluorescent lighting with soft low-wattage lighting. Pheromone diffusers for dogs and cats can also be added along with soothing music (**Fig. 2**).[6] Joshua Leeds, a psychoacoustic expert has documented how music can help to calm animal patients.[7] Depending on the practitioner and staff's preferences, candles, wind chimes, and a water fountain feature can also modify the room into a more peaceful retreat. Make sure there is comfortable seating for the pet owners and a restful space for the pet. The temperature of the room should be adjusted to suit the comfort of the pet. Some hospitals may have peaceful outdoor gardens or areas where the euthanasia could also take place. A summary of hospital environmental enrichment options is found in **Box 5**.

Another nonpharmacologic intervention to improve the euthanasia experience is taking control over hospital appointment logistics. A summary of logistic options is found in **Box 6**. It is beneficial to have proactive scheduling during quiet times of

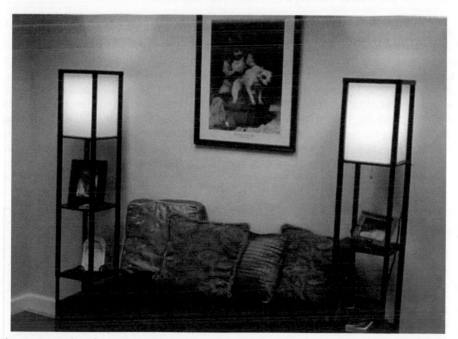

Fig. 2. Example of a proper hospital environment. Note the lighting and comfortable seating.

Box 5
Hospital environmental enrichment options

Nonslip floor

Use of pheromones

Soft lighting

Comfortable temperature

Comfortable seating

Soothing music

Candles

Quiet environment

Water feature, fountain

Wind chimes

Peaceful outdoor yard or garden areas

---

the day (before or after routine appointments are completed) and allowing an extended appointment time to ensure the pet owner has ample time with their pet before and after the euthanasia. It is encouraged that during the appointment time the hospital staff be mindful and quiet in respect for the death of the pet. Various codes are used in multidoctor practices to alert that a euthanasia is in progress. These codes include placement of a special flag on the comfort or examination room door, turning on a special light, or playing specific music. The staff should provide considerate aftercare of the pet's body treating it carefully and respectfully.

Set up the home environment

Before euthanasia, a personalized plan should include helping the caretaker set up an area in their home to care for their pet until the appropriate time for euthanasia or a hospice-assisted natural death occurs. Depending on the pet's needs and personality, either a quiet location or a social location might be appropriate. It is important for many pets to be part of the normal family activities so accommodations to meet these needs should be a priority. Nonslip flooring with good traction should be available to minimize the risk of falls for pets that can still ambulate and stairways should be blocked to prevent falls for pets that are unstable. For pets that are allowed on furniture or beds, low incline steps or ramps should be provided. All locations where the pet may reside should have access to water so they do not have to go to another location for

---

Box 6
Hospital appointment logistic options

Schedule during quiet times of day

Schedule adequate, extended appointment time

Provide a mindful and quiet environment

Allow pet owner to spend ample time with their pet

Encourage memorialization

Provide respectful aftercare

---

hydration. Elevated feeders or hand feeding should be provided for pets that have a posture problem making the lowering of their heads difficult. Litter box access should be made easier by moving it closer to the cat, lowering the sides, and increasing the size of the box. Some cats can learn to use a hygiene pad sprinkled with kitty litter instead of a litter box. Thermal comfort should be adjusted for the individual. Pets that are chilled need added warmth but care must be taken because debilitated pets do not thermoregulate well and often cannot move away from a heat source. If an outdoor pet cannot be brought inside, care must be given to protect it from temperature extremes in addition to fly strike in the warmer months and frostbite or freezing when it is cold.

The environment during the last hours of life should be made as peaceful as possible for the pet. At the time of euthanasia, the pet owner may consider letting the pet choose its favorite spot. Even outside the hospital, the use of pheromones and music therapy may provide additional comfort.

Euthanasia logistics
The personalized plan helps to organize where the euthanasia will take place and who will be in attendance for the event. Pet owners may choose to have the euthanasia performed in the veterinary hospital, at home, or at a different location (in the pet's favorite place) (**Fig. 3**). It is helpful to plan who will be in attendance. This may include family, friends, and neighbors that were close to the pet. Another often overlooked aspect that can be part of the euthanasia process for pets with an appetite is the offering of special treats to the pet as part of the process (**Fig. 4**).

Preplanning final arrangements
There are also nonpharmaceutical benefits in providing information about final arrangement options as part of the personalized plan. The practitioner should provide resources and conversation with the pet owner that includes final arrangement options

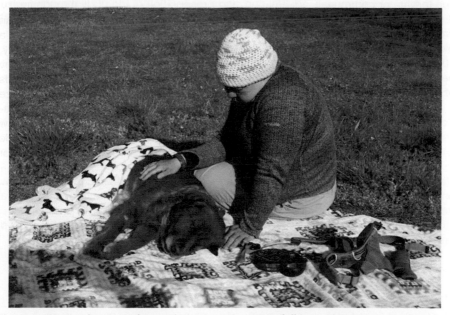

Fig. 3. Patient and owner after euthanasia sitting peacefully together on a lawn outside a clinic.

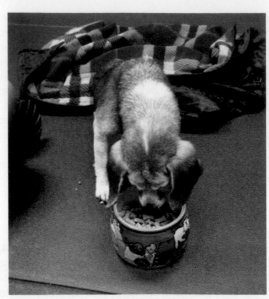

Fig. 4. Karma eating from the clinic cookie jar while the pre-euthanasia sedative takes effect.

for their pet so that the care they were receiving in life is reflective in the thoughtful choices at the time of death. In human medicine, advanced care planning discussion has also been shown to significantly reduce symptoms of post-traumatic stress, anxiety, and depression in surviving family members.[8]

Discussion about the final arrangements might include the choices of burial, cremation (private or communal), aquamation, and preservation of the body through freeze drying. If burial on private property is chosen, it is important to be familiar with local ordinances and what standards are necessary for a proper burial. When legal, examples of some guidelines include: identify and avoid buried utilities, provide at least a 100-foot separation from wells and waterways, a 4-foot separation should be made between the ground water and a burial, avoid areas that flood, and provide a minimum of 3 feet of soil on top of the pet's body to prevent scavenging.[9]

Pet owners may appreciate knowing that memorial service options are appropriate. Some might choose to invite friends and family together even before the euthanasia to celebrate the pet's life and be able to say final good-byes before the euthanasia. Others might choose to have a visitation or wake after the pet's passing to pay tribute to their loved-one. During these times, there are various ways to memorialize the pet's life through art forms and oral tributes. Some considerations include making a paw print or nose print, taking a clipping of hair, creating jewelry, planting flowers or a tree, painting a picture, making a stepping stone or personalized marker, reading a story, creating poetry, or making a donation of time or money in behalf of the loved one to a charity (**Fig.5**).

Box 7 provides a personalized care plan checklist that ensures that no part of the planning is overlooked.

Step 4: Organize and Carry Out the Euthanasia

The fourth step includes carrying out the personalized euthanasia plan that has been previously outlined. Besides having the equipment and drugs to carry out the

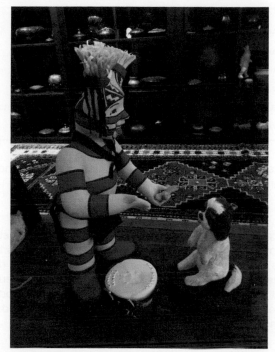

Fig. 5. Pottery consignment by artist Kathleen Wall to honor Little Bit.

euthanasia as described in Step 3, it is important to make sure all details are in place to carry out the euthanasia. For example, the practitioner should be prepared for the location of the euthanasia and dress appropriately if the euthanasia is conducted outdoors.

Tips to help practitioners provide the best euthanasia include being on time with house call appointments and being respectful of the pet owner's home. Appointments for euthanasia in the veterinary clinic should also be punctual. After euthanasia, examples of nonpharmaceutical efforts to make the experience easier for the pet owner are helping with the closure of eyes at the time of death, conducting necessary hygiene, and carefully preparing the body to be moved by supporting the pet's head and neck.

Step 5: Emotional Support During the Care Process and After the Death of the Pet

Even though this step is listed as fifth, it is important that the veterinarian and staff begin to support the caretaker when a pet is first diagnosed with a chronic or life-limiting disease. In addition to the veterinary staff, social workers, psychologists, and bereavement counselors can help provide emotional support before, during, and after the euthanasia process. If a practice does not employ a multidisciplinary team, this care may be outsourced. Arrangements can be made with these nonveterinary support professionals who have an interest in animal welfare to help the family. If the team uses outside spiritual support, it is important for such professionals to respect the cultural traditions and spiritual beliefs of the pet owner.

After the death of a pet, bereavement counseling should last as long as necessary. In human hospice the bereavement counseling may last for more than 1 year. When needed, the veterinary staff should be able to recommend services to help pet owners grieve the loss of a pet. Also veterinarians and staff should recognize and be able to

---

Box 7
The personalized care plan checklist

Arrange for 24-hour care

Offer treatment and euthanasia options that match psychosocial views

Provide the proper hospital setting or comfortable home environment

Outline euthanasia logistics: identify where the euthanasia will take place and who will attend

Preplanning final details

---

help surviving pets that are suffering with behavioral changes secondary to the death of a companion animal.

SUMMARY

Using a hospice care plan or implementing common tips used by veterinary hospice/palliative care providers helps the family, practitioner, and support staff, but most importantly, helps to ensure that the pet is comfortable before and during the euthanasia process. These nonpharmaceutical methods to improve the euthanasia experience are as equally important as the drugs used to carry out a good euthanasia and are also cost effective. The integration of pharmaceutical and nonpharmaceutical methods is paramount in providing a good death.

REFERENCES

1. Herbert R, Prigerson H, Schultz R, et al. Preparing caregivers for the death of a loved one: a theoretical framework and suggestions for future research. J Palliat Med 2006;9:1164–9.
2. Shearer T. Hospice and palliative care. In: Gaynor J, Muir W, editors. Handbook of veterinary pain management. 2nd edition. St Louis (MO): Mosby; 2010. p. 590–6.
3. Shearer T. Delivery systems of veterinary hospice and palliative care. Vet Clin North Am Small Anim Pract 2011;41:499–505.
4. Borden LJ, Adams CL, Bonnett BN, et al. Comparison of veterinarian and client perceptions of communication during euthanasia discussions. J Am Vet Med Assoc 2019;254(9):1073–85.
5. Leary S, Underwood W, Anthony R, et al. AVMA guidelines for the euthanasia of animals: 2013 edition. Available at: https://www.avma.org/KB/Policies/Documents/euthanasia.pdf. Accessed January 12, 2018.
6. Kim YM, Lee JK, Abdel A, et al. Efficacy of dog appeasing pheromone (DAP) for ameliorating separation-related behavioral signs in hospitalized dogs. Can Vet J 2010;4:380–4.
7. Wells DL, Graham L, Hepper PG. The influence of auditory stimulation on the behavior of dogs housed in a rescue shelter. Anim Welf 2002;11:385–93.
8. Detering K, Hancock A, Reade M, et al. The impact of advance care planning on end of life care in elderly patients: randomized controlled trial. BMJ 2010;340: c1345.
9. Cooney K. In-home pet euthanasia techniques. 2nd edition. Loveland (CO): Cooney Publishing; 2016. p. 112–4.

The Role of the Veterinary Technician in End-of-Life Care

Kelly Carter, RVT

KEYWORDS

- Palliative care veterinary technician • Hospice care veterinary technician
- End-of-life care • Euthanasia • Nursing care

KEY POINTS

- The veterinary technician plays an important role serving as a conduit among the veterinarian, client, and patient.
- The veterinary technician helps to carry out important aspects of nursing care to maintain quality of life.
- Client education about end of life and euthanasia can be delegated to the veterinary technician.
- The efforts of a veterinary technician may reduce caregiver burden for the client and veterinarian.

The role of the veterinary technician in addressing end-of-life care in veterinary medicine has a profound impact on the quality of life during the final days by providing much needed palliative care. "Palliative care is a philosophy and a unique set of care processes that aim to enhance quality of life for people with a life-limiting condition and to provide support for their families. Part of this is providing high quality end-of-life care to help ensure that people can have a 'good death', ideally in the place of their choosing."[1] Now is the time for the same care and philosophy to be applied to elder animals with debilitating illness and their families. Palliative care is also appropriate for pets of any age who have an illness that is life limiting.

As stated by the International Association of Animal Hospice and Palliative Medicine's Guidelines for Recommended Practices in Animal Palliative Care (2017)[2], "Palliation is defined as relieving or soothing the symptoms of a disease or disorder at any stage of an illness. Animal palliative care guides animals' caregivers (their human family members or owners) in making plans for living well based on the animals' needs and concerns and on the caregivers' goals for care." There

4 Paws Farewell: Mobile Pet Hospice, Palliative Care and Home Euthanasia, Asheville, NC, USA
E-mail address: kellyc4paws@gmail.com

Vet Clin Small Anim 50 (2020) 639–645
https://doi.org/10.1016/j.cvsm.2019.12.012
0195-5616/20/© 2020 Elsevier Inc. All rights reserved.

are many studies on how effective human hospice/palliative care is beneficial to the patient and family members.[3,4] Animal palliative care is being recognized as a more viable option for end-of-life care. This article highlights the pivotal role veterinarian technicians can play in veterinary palliative and hospice care. Because hospice is a form of palliative care, the term veterinary palliative care is used.

The support of the palliative care veterinary technician is important after a life-limiting diagnosis or geriatric decline has been identified and discussed with a veterinarian. The veterinary technician is the communication conduit between client and doctor and doctor and "patient" (pet). At times, the palliative care veterinary technician is responsible for explaining how the patient ("pet")/client relationship will change regarding what to expect throughout end-of-life care. Setting the tone for open communication with the client addresses medical and emotional needs during this delicate time.

Often the palliative care veterinary technician is able to see signs in the patient that the client does not notice. This is not because the client is neglecting the pet, but rather certain subtle signs are not obvious. The caregiver does not notice how much they are compensating for the patient's inabilities. The palliative care veterinary technician is able to give her or his perception of medical symptoms and explain them to the client in a way that they will understand. Such signs include: monitoring weight, body language, mobility, interactive behavior, and signs of pain or anxiety. Not only are signs based on visual appearances, they are also based on the natural body cycles of dying and decompensation. Chronic inappetence is a common problem during palliative care. The palliative care veterinary technician is helpful by giving a list of palatable foods options (Appendix 1).

Monitoring resting respiration rates, heart rates, and capillary refill times gives the veterinarian a daily or weekly update on the patient's vital signs. The veterinary technician can also teach the client to monitor certain vital signs at home. The veterinary technician can monitor blood pressure as needed, in the home setting if applicable, to avoid the unnecessary health complication of untreated hypertension. Blood pressures obtained in the home setting are thought to be more reliable. The veterinary technician is always keeping the veterinarian informed to continue a desired level of analgesia, comfort, and welfare.

In the hospital setting, the palliative care veterinary technician can help see decline or progress because of treatment with medications, the effects of implemented prophylactics, and the influence of the hospital environment on a daily basis. If the patient is in-home palliative care, they are generally monitored on a weekly basis. Having a veterinary technician who is knowledgeable about common palliative care disease processes is valuable to the client and the veterinarian, and is crucial for elder pets. The palliative care veterinary technician should be familiar with all medications used and their side effects. Using the veterinary technician saves time for the doctor and gives the caregiver a known relationship they can depend on, often decreasing the caregiver's burden. Veterinary caregiver burden has recently been identified and has been associated with distress in pet owners caring for a sick pet.[5] "The goal of proper and effective geriatric pet care is to enhance the quality of life for the pet and the owners, empower them to properly care for their pet during this delicate life phase, and maintain the strength of human-animal bond."[6–14]

In addition to the client, the palliative care veterinary technician often helps to keep the patient clean and comfortable. Showing clients how to implement this into their normal routine, when at home, is beneficial for geriatric pets. As they get older they bathe themselves less, frequently become incontinent, and often acquire hot spots or bed sores. Educating clients on ways to prepare for such occurrences reduces the patient's discomfort and gives the client proactive duties to which to adhere (Appendix 2).

Stress in traveling, having compromised mobility, and reacting to unknown environments are avoided by having medical services provided in the home. The mobile palliative veterinary technician can give subcutaneous fluids and injections, offer ideas on how to stabilize the companion's mobility, and provide a support system for the caregiver.

Frequently, the veterinary technician sees the hospice/palliative care pet over time, and can offer different ideas for mobility assistance as mobility declines. Veterinary technicians are adept at measuring pets for assistance devices or applying mobility aids, such as toe grips (**Figs. 1–3**).

Applications available to patient	Environmental Applications available	Other recommendations per DVM
ToeGrips and shave paws	Raised food and water dish	Laser therapy
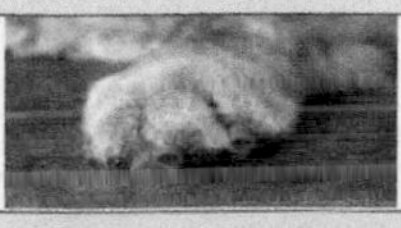	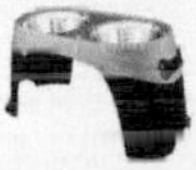	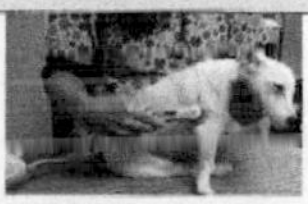
Help'em up Harness	Yoga mats or carpet runners	Acupuncture
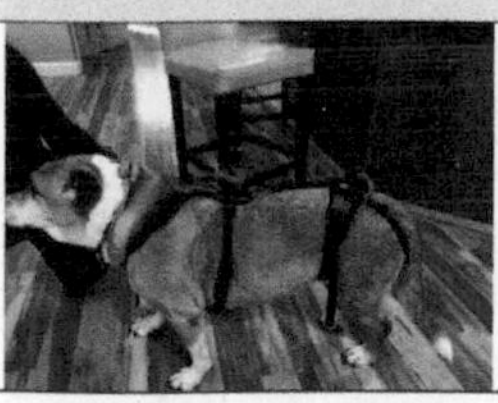	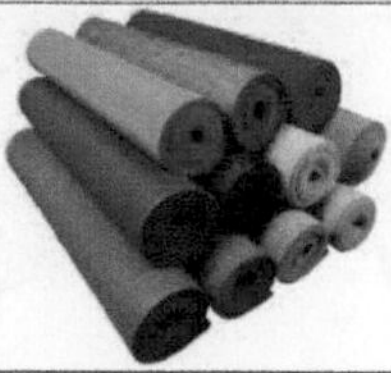	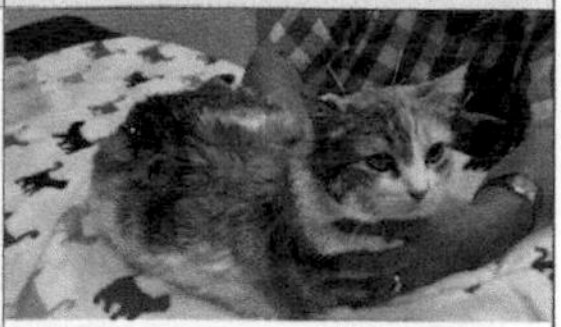
	Steps and levels for older cats	
	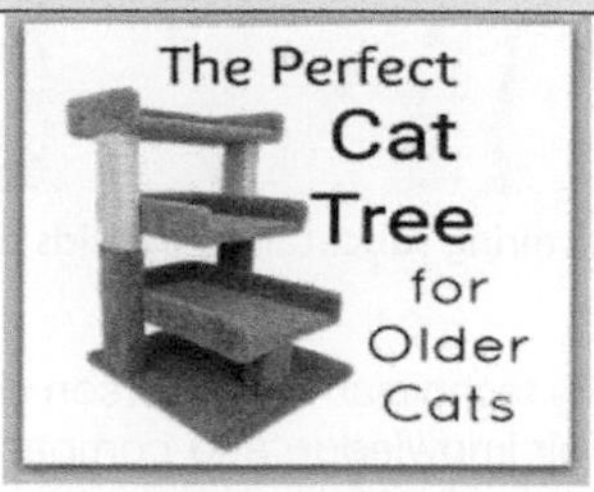	

Fig. 1. Mobility aids.

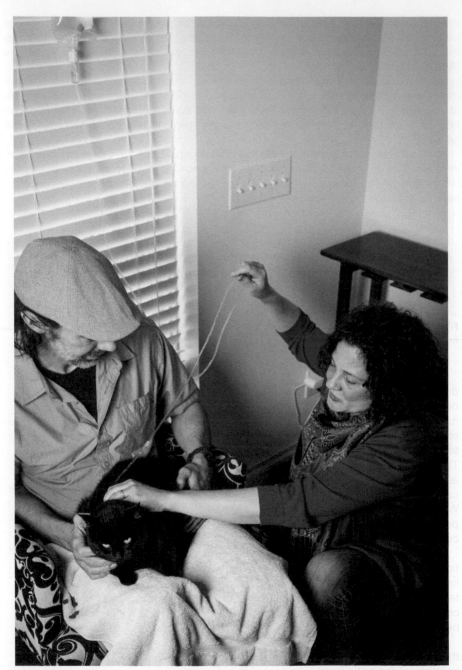

Fig. 2. Kelly Carter, RVT administering subcutaneous fluids to Roxy while Roxy is in the lap of her owner, Michael Mercier.

The palliative care veterinary technician is the person who daily, or weekly, gives reassurance to the client with their knowledge and compassion during this unpredictable time. The veterinary technician is often the reminder that palliative care is about quality, compassion, and dignity in living with an illness and not necessarily about living longer.

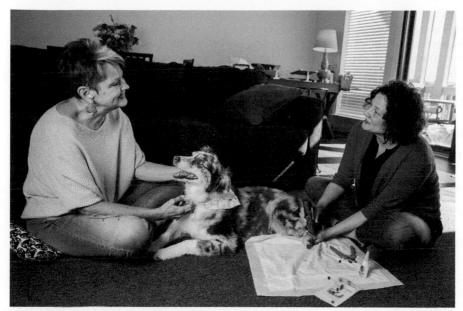

Fig. 3. Kelly Carter, RVT applying ToeGrips® to Honor in her home with her owner Patricia Robertson. (*Courtesy of* Dr. Buzby's Innovations, LLC, Beaufort, SC.)

In human hospice, a social worker and/or clergy member, is often available if one desires or the family chooses to elect to have them present. In veterinary medicine, neither home-based palliative care/hospice services or those provided in the clinic have reached the level of having a grief counselor or clergy readily available on staff. Emotional support is crucial for the caregiver. The palliative care veterinary technician becomes the social support for the client when visits are frequent. The client often relies on them for processing the end-of-life experience and serving as a sounding board for the emotions the caregiver is experiencing. If or when this care is provided, the patient's family should have access to relevant pamphlets, Web sites, and/or business cards. The palliative care veterinary technician is the person to relay those resources, including pet loss support groups and grief counselors.

Often, clients experience "white coat" syndrome. They feel as though their questions are "not worth the doctors time" or are too financially focused. Clients should know the financial information to make the best decision for their family. The veterinary technician with whom the client has been communicating is often the one to explain cost, billing, and services administered. Home palliative care, where available, should be presented as an alternate option to in-hospital care.

The veterinary technician may also help facilitate euthanasia logistics and details that may include the preferred location of the euthanasia and details about the handling of the pet's body. The technician should make sure the pet and the family are comfortable and that there are plenty of towels, blankets, and waterproof pads. If in a clinic setting they should make sure that all of the staff are aware there is a euthanasia in process by notifying them or using a code of some sort (special music, a ribbon on the door knob, a special light turned on). In a clinic situation, the veterinary technician may stay with the client before, during, and after the euthanasia.

The role of the veterinary technician in end-of-life care is vital and multifaceted. Their role is ever-changing, using human hospice care as a model to better understand the importance of palliative care in animals. We know the outcome is a natural death or euthanasia. How the patient and client experience the time beforehand, however, leaves a lasting impression. Veterinary technicians have unique skills, talents, and perspective that can greatly influence this time by helping to enhance and maintain the human-animal bond and provide compassionate, dignified care.

DISCLOSURE

The author has nothing to disclose.

ACKNOWLEDGMENTS

Pictures provided by Caren Harris, caren@carenharrisphotography.com.

REFERENCES

1. Kassalainen S, Ploeg J, McAiney C, et al. Role of the nurse practitioner in providing palliative care in long-term care homes. Int J Palliat Nurs 2013; 19(10):477–85.
2. August K, Cooney K, Hendrix L et al. Guidelines for recommended practices in animal hospice and palliative care. 2017. Available at: https://www.iaahpc. org/images/2017_IAAHPC_Animal_Hospice_and_Palliative_Care_Guidelines. pdf. Accessed September 1, 2019.
3. Cherlin EJ, Brewster AL, Curry LA, et al. Interventions for reducing hospital readmission rates: the role of hospice and palliative care. Am J Hosp Palliat Care 2017;34(8):748–53.
4. Yennurajalingam S, Urbauer DL, Casper K, et al. Impact of palliative care consultation team on cancer-related symptoms in advanced cancer patients referred to an outpatient support care clinic. J Pain Symptom Manage 2011;41(1):49–56.
5. Spitznagel MB, Jacobson DM, Cox MD, et al. Caregiver burden in owners of sick companion animals: a cross sectional observational study. Vet Rec 2017; 181(12):321.
6. Gardner M. Caring for clients around end-of-life care. In: Proceedings 2018 New York State Veterinary Conference. Ithaca, NY, 2008. pp. 1-5. Available at: https://www.vin.com/doc/?id=8760750 [Accessed September 15, 2019]
7. Hendrix L. Tech Time!. In: Proceedings International Association of Animal Hospice and Palliative Care Conference. San Diego, CA, 2015. pp 1-5. Available at: URL: https://www.vin.com/doc/?id=7360488 [Accessed September 15, 2019]
8. Siddens AD. Rehabilitation for the veterinary technician. Veterinary Team Brief; 2014. Available at: https://www.cliniciansbrief.com/article/rehabilitation-techniques-veterinary-technician. Accessed September 15, 2019.
9. Good J. Role of the technician within the oncology service. In: Proceedings Western Veterinary Conference. Las Vegas, NV, 2008. p.1–5. Available at: https://www.vin.com/doc/?id=3862082. Accessed September 15, 2019.
10. Shaffran N. Pain management: the veterinary technician's perspective. Vet Clin Small Anim 2008;38:1415–28.
11. Glajchen M, Goehring A. The family meeting palliative care: role of the oncology nurse. Semin Oncol Nurs 2017;33(5):489–97.

12. Arnaert A, Wainwright M. Providing care and sharing expertise: reflections of nurse specialists in palliative home care. Palliat Support Care 2009;7(3): 35–64.
13. Rosser M, King L. Transition experiences of qualified nurses moving into hospice nursing. J Adv Nurs 2003;43(2):111–217.
14. Mok E, Chiu PC. Nurse-patient relationships in palliative care. J Adv Nurs 2004; 48(5):475–83.

APPENDIX 1: FOODS FOR INAPPETENCE OR TO DISGUISE MEDICATION IN

- Braunschweiger (also known as liverwurst)
- Cream cheese
- Hot dogs/Vienna sausage
- Canned pate cat food
- Canned squeeze cheese
- Lunch meat
- Canned chicken, salmon or tripe
- Peanut butter
- Marshmallows
- Pill pockets

Other Ideas Regarding Food

Use butter to seal in the flavor of the capsule/tablet and then wrap in a slice of deli meat or softened cheese

Avoid creating an association between medication and the food used to hide the medication:

- Offer several small tastes of the food (medication free), then the food with the medication, then more medication-free food.
- Offer the food at times other than when medicating expressing a positive invitation with: "here's a treat", "here's a cookie"

Vary the foods used to deliver the medication.

Avoid touching the food with hands that have touched the medication.

- With clean hands make a small patty of the food
- Place or have someone else place the medication in the patty
- Wrap the food around the medication with clean hands

To increase palatability and to tempt picky appetites:

- Microwave the food to just above room temperature to release more smells and mimic prey temperature
- Add flavoring ingredients such as small amounts of some of the foods above, grilled chicken or beef or their juices, or low sodium chicken broth
- Small frequent meals offered in a quiet space with lots of human coaxing (hand-feeding) or sometimes with a slight amount of competition from dog siblings (compiled by Mary Lummis, DVM)

APPENDIX 2: KEEPING PATIENTS CLEAN AND COMFORTABLE

- Face washing with a warm cloth: feels good and promotes bathing
- Clipping nails to prevent getting hung up on materials
- Have non scented wipes available, use warm water to soak up in the wipes to keep patient clean
- Keep a "sanitary clip" to prevent urine and feces from adhering to the fur
- Gentle brushing

Case Reports
Challenging Euthanasia Cases

Lauren Orvin, DVM, CHPV*

KEYWORDS

- Euthanasia • Oral pre-sedation protocols • Aggression • Respiratory distress
- Alternative routes of administration

KEY POINTS

- Maintain safety for the practitioner, staff, and owners at every step in the euthanasia process.
- Be prepared with several options for medications and routes of administration for euthanasia presedation and for euthanasia solutions.
- Client education is of great importance in the euthanasia setting, particularly when deviating from an initial plan or from the family's previous experiences.
- A practitioner's understanding of clients' expectations about euthanasia is helpful in guiding them through the process.

INTRODUCTION

There are many factors that influence a family's decision for euthanasia, including prognosis, cost of treatment, the pet's quality of life, and the impact on the family in caring for an ill pet. Owners face the challenge of making the decision for euthanasia, whereas practitioners face the challenge of providing a peaceful and humane euthanasia to the pet and family. The following cases explore the challenges surrounding euthanasia of an unpredictably aggressive pet, an obese pet, and a pet with respiratory disease. Each case required improvisation, problem-solving skills, and open communication with the family.

CASE ONE: HOME EUTHANASIA—UNPREDICTABLE AGGRESSION

The reality of behavioral euthanasia is a complicated and challenging subject for both veterinarians and pet owners. Aggression in particular is one of the more common reasons for behavioral euthanasia or relinquishment to shelters. There are many factors that influence a family's decision to euthanize for behavioral problems. These may

Lowcountry Pet Hospice and Home Euthanasia
* 1099 Sugar Hill Drive, Moncks Corner, SC.
E-mail address: dr.orvin@lowcountrypethospice.com

Vet Clin Small Anim 50 (2020) 647–652
https://doi.org/10.1016/j.cvsm.2019.12.013
0195-5616/20/© 2019 Elsevier Inc. All rights reserved.

include safety, duration and escalation of the problem, predictability of the behavior, and expense related to attempting treatment options. Guilt and shame can complicate the decision-making process further. Regardless of the influencing factors, veterinarians are faced with the logistical task of humanely euthanizing pets that are a safety risk.

Axel was a 6-year-old, male neutered, English bulldog (38 kg) whose owners reached out after progressively aggressive behaviors culminated in a severe bite to the owner requiring medical attention. It was discovered that he had become increasingly more aggressive over the past few months, but the initial aggression started several years before after experiencing head trauma that left him unconscious for several minutes. As a result of his aggression, the pet had not recently been vaccinated against rabies and was placed under a 10-day home quarantine, which was nearing its end.

On initial phone contact with the owner, he expressed concerns over the procedure of sedation prior to euthanasia, considering the family was unable to leash the pet any longer without aggressive behaviors. All avenues to have the pet removed from the home, including local animal control and animal shelters, had been exhausted and they felt that home euthanasia was the only option. The family also expressed significant guilt over the decision to euthanize and that they felt they were no longer safe with him in the home. His behavior had escalated to the point of becoming reactive to any interactions, including attempts to place a collar or leash on him or to pet his head. Injectable sedation was not deemed safe for the practitioner or the family to attempt, and the decision was made to administer oral sedation during the first appointment and monitor his response before proceeding with additional injectable sedatives prior to euthanasia. In discussing a strategy for sedation, oral sedatives ideally would provide enough sedation for the practitioner to safely administer injectable medications to achieve deep sedation prior to euthanasia, with the goal being safety of everyone involved at every step in the process.[1] The owner felt that the pet would readily accept oral medications and inquired about attempting oral sedation and, at the practitioner's discretion, proceeding with euthanasia at the first appointment, because the pet's presence in the home was causing increasing stress to the family. Attempting euthanasia during the first appointment was agreed on, depending on the pet's response to the sedatives.

The pet would be fasted the morning of the appointment to allow for increased success.

On the day of the initial appointment, Axel was quarantined to the dining area with the use of baby gates to block the open doorways and direct access to the fenced in back yard. This is where he had been kept for the prior week due to the owner's concerns for safety.

The practitioner's arrival did not create any increased stress for him, and in fact he was calmer than usual. Oral gabapentin capsules (100 mg/kg) and crushed acepromazine tablets (10 mg/kg) were administered in a small amount of food. After 15 minutes, Axel was ataxic, but made attempts to get up and walk a little ways before lying back down. After an additional 30 minutes, he lay down just next to the gated area in the kitchen and was amenable to detomidine gel administration, oral transmucosal (7.6 mg).[2] He got up 1 more time before lying down in his bed and began snoring loudly. An additional 15 minutes time was given before attempting to administer injectable tiletamine hydrochloride/zolazepam hydrochloride (3 mg/kg).[3] Two attempts were made to give the subcutaneous injection, but the pet became aggressive again, despite the administration of significant oral and transmucosal sedatives. Thus, further attempts were not made on that day.

Communications were maintained with the family over the next 2 days to ensure the pet recovered from the sedatives administered. The family reported he was sleepy and eating some. The decision was made to regroup and attempt a different type of oral protocol 3 days after the initial visit, when the pet was eating more reliably. The pet was to be fasted; as before, the home would not be entered until he was sedated to prevent any additional stress, and an assistant was brought along at the second appointment.

The following meal was prepared for Axel on the front porch on arrival:

1. With gloved hands, 100 mg of dry tiletamine hydrochloride/zolazepam hydrochloride was removed from the bottle and broken into smaller pieces and placed in a single meatball of raw hamburger.
2. Acepromazine tablets (approximately 800 mg) were crushed and mixed into 2 additional raw hamburger meatballs.
3. Pentobarbital sodium/phenytoin sodium solution (approximately 3000 mg) was injected into several empty gel capsules and wrapped in cheese slices.

The entire meal was coated in ketchup to mask any bitterness. The meal was offered to Axel, which he accepted with encouragement, and he consumed the entirety of tiletamine hydrochloride/zolazepam hydrochloride, acepromazine, and approximately 1500 mg of the pentobarbital/phenytoin capsules.

The owner was instructed to check on the pet every 15 minutes while veterinary staff remained outside to avoid unnecessary stress and stimulation. After 30 minutes, the pet was lying down and no longer attempting to get up and walk around. After 45 minutes he was no longer responsive (head/ear/eye movements) to sound. Finally, after 60 minutes and significantly longer than anticipated, the pet was not responsive to touch. Due to previous experience with sedation and reactivity, a blanket was placed across the pet to provide another layer of protection to the practitioner. No response was elicited. Pentobarbital sodium (3 mL/4.5 kg body weight) was administered as an intraperitoneal injection.[4,5] This choice was made versus attempting an intravenous (IV) catheter because of the ease and quickness of administration. After 30 minutes, however, the pet's respiratory rate was persistent and an attempt was made to place an IV catheter in the lateral saphenous vein, which was successful. Pentobarbital solution (1.5 mL/4.5 kg body weight) was administered and the pet passed away immediately after injection.[3]

Axel's case demonstrates the logistical hurdles for safe, humane euthanasia in an aggressive and unpredictable pet, particularly in the home setting. In these situations, it is easy to shift into a goal-oriented approach of safely euthanizing the pet, but it also is important to approach these cases with patience. This includes the ability to regroup, reschedule the visit if necessary, and change medications accordingly, even resorting to off-label usage, as was necessary in this case. Demonstrating patience and persistence in the care of the pet and family is needed to achieve the ultimate goal of a peaceful passing.

CASE TWO: HOME EUTHANASIA—RESPIRATORY DISTRESS

Pets with respiratory disease present unique challenges to euthanasia both logistically and in terms of a family's experience. Often, these cases are of an urgent or emergent nature, which creates an additional level of anxiety for the patient, the family, and the veterinary provider. Creating a calm euthanasia experience helps providers honor the bond between pet and family. Abigail was an 11-year-old, female spayed, pit bull mix (18 kg). She was diagnosed by fine-needle aspiration with a suspected thyroid neoplasia approximately 18 months before entering hospice care. She had survived her prognosis significantly longer than anticipated and initially was receiving prednisone (0.5 mg/kg) and cannabidiol oil (unknown dose) as palliative care through her primary care veterinarian. In the few weeks before euthanasia, her respiratory effort increased (including more abdominal effort and use of accessory muscles), the noise of respiration had become louder and harsher, and her bark had changed. During the short time she was in hospice care, her respiratory effort continued to become more laborious and her ability to swallow declined to an inability to eat, prompting election of euthanasia.

The initial plan was to give injectable acepromazine (0.25 mg/kg) to reduce the anxiety associated with her increased respiratory efforts and injectable butorphanol (0.25 mg/kg) as a sedative[6] to facilitate IV catheter placement and allow for sodium pentobarbital administration. Dexmedetomidine was excluded from the initial plan because of the possibility of bradycardia and apnea.[3] When attempting to give the subcutaneous injection, however, Abigail became fearful and noncooperative, causing her respiratory rate to increase. During consultation with the owner, it was decided injectable presedation was not in the pet's best interest and a plan for a 2-step presedation before euthanasia was devised. The risk for respiratory distress was discussed with the additional sedation, but parameters that would be closely monitored (respiratory rate, effort, noise, and any reflexive/agonal breathing) and preparations for quick intervention were explained thoroughly. Oral detomidine gel (approximately 2 mg/m²)[2] was utilized to allow for a less stressful first sedation. Once Abigail was mildly sedated, the additional doses of acepromazine (0.25 mg/kg)[3] and butorphanol (0.25 mg/kg)[3] were administered as a single subcutaneous injection to achieve a deeper level of sedation for IV catheter placement. Preparations for a quick intervention at the beginning of the sedation process were organized, having all necessary tools (butterfly IV catheter, opened; syringe of saline to flush IV catheter; sodium pentobarbital solution, drawn up and accessible; hair clippers; and so forth)[5] close at hand should Abigail experience respiratory distress. Although her respiratory rate decreased with sedation, her respiratory noise and inspiratory efforts began to increase significantly, causing concern for possible obstruction. The owner was gently informed that the veterinarians should proceed with euthanasia. Because this had been discussed with the owner during presedation, a lengthy explanation was not needed and the IV catheter was placed and sodium pentobarbital (1 mL/4.5 kg body weight)[3] was administered without incident, and Abigail passed away with minimal respiratory distress. Two agonal respirations were noticed after her passing.[7] Despite the beginning signs of respiratory distress, the owner was grateful that the veterinarians did not proceed with the initial plan of approaching Abigail with injectable sedation because it caused her distress. The addition of transmucosal detomidine hydrochloride gel prior to injectable sedation allowed her to be more relaxed for the subcutaneous injection. Ideally, agonal respirations would not have occurred; however, the owner felt informed about the possible risk and causes for her observations. Ultimately, she expressed a sense of peace about the experience for herself and for Abigail.

CASE THREE: HOME EUTHANASIA—CHALLENGING INTRAVENOUS ACCESS

In some cases, a pet's disease process or body condition makes IV catheter placement too difficult or impossible. This deviates from what clients may expect or what they have experienced with previous euthanasia experiences. The challenge presents itself in the comfort level of the veterinarian to move beyond traditional routes of administration and the family's acceptance of these deviations. The challenge is met when the veterinarian is prepared and can appropriately educate the family in the event that those methods have to be utilized.

An elderly woman living alone owned Heidi, a 14-year-old, female spayed, standard dachshund (25 kg). Her previous in-home euthanasia experiences included presedation and IV catheter placement for administration of euthanasia solutions. Heidi was diagnosed with hyperadrenocorticism and hypothyroidism, but treatment had been declined. The decision to euthanize Heidi was made based on her poor and declining mobility and her severe urinary incontinence. In general, Heidi had no bladder control and was constantly polyuric and polydipsic, creating a level of nursing care greater than the owner's abilities. Heidi also was morbidly obese, with a body condition score of 9/9.

On presentation in the home, Heidi struggled to move around on the carpeted floors and exhibited an increased respiratory rate and effort when ambulating. There also was evidence of urine and urine staining along her hind limbs.

During Heidi's assessment, it was discussed that due to her body condition, sedation may take longer or require additional dosing along with the potential challenges that her breed conformation may present, including IV access.

She initially was sedated with acepromazine (0.25 mg/kg),[3] butorphanol (0.25 mg/kg),[3] and dexmedetomidine (4 µg/kg)[3] subcutaneously; however, after 15 minutes, she was still responsive to sound and touch. The initial sedative presumably was slowly absorbed due to injection into subcutaneous fat and, in the interest of time for the pet and family, additional acepromazine and butorphanol were administered intramuscularly at the previously stated dose. An additional 10 minutes passed and the pet's palpebral reflexes were diminished to nearly absent and her deep pain reflex was entirely absent.

Attempts to place a butterfly catheter in the lateral saphenous vein, cephalic vein, accessory cephalic vein, and dorsal pedal veins were unsuccessful. Due to the pet's obesity, underlying medical condition, and anatomic confirmation, placement was deemed not possible. At that time, alternative means for euthanasia were discussed with the owner.[3] The process of intraperitoneal injection was explained: simply that the vessels within the belly would allow the medication to be absorbed slowly, taking approximately 20 minutes to 30 minutes or more. It was explained that she was asleep and the injection would not be painful or stressful for her. The owner was encouraged to continue to pet and talk to her just as before.

Sodium pentobarbital (3 mL/4.5 kg body weight body weight)[5] was administered intraperitoneal[4] with an 18-g, 1.5-in needle and the patient was monitored closely. After 30 minutes, her heart rate and respiratory rates remained stable. Because her vital signs were stable, there was concern that the medication may have been injected into abdominal fat, thus slowing or inhibiting absorption.

The decision was made to help her pass on by giving an intracardiac injection. For reassurance, it was demonstrated that the pet's deep pain reflexes were absent on multiple extremities and even her palpebral reflexes were absent at this point.

An additional dose of sodium pentobarbital (1 mL/4.5 kg body weight) H[3] was administered intracardiac[4] using an 18-g, 1.5-in needle. The practitioner's body was positioned such that the injection into the pericardium was shielded from the owner's view. A small amount of blood was aspirated into the syringe prior to injection to ensure proper placement into the heart. The pet passed almost instantly with administration of the entire intracardiac dose.

Heidi's case exemplifies the multiple options veterinarians have at their disposal for humane euthanasia. It also demonstrates the necessity of communicating challenges that may arise during the euthanasia process in a calm and confident manner. Setting realistic expectations with a family in these unusual situations helps them to be confident in a veterinarian's ability to improvise the approach, if needed.

After Heidi's passing, the owner and her neighbor expressed their thankfulness for patience and persistence despite the challenges Heidi's case presented. Education during the process of euthanasia and a gentle demeanor helped Heidi's owner to be comfortable despite the deviations from the initial plan.

SUMMARY

Decisions for euthanasia are as varied as pets, and, as such, challenges often arise. The practitioner's focus always must be to meet those challenges with patience and provide a gentle and humane experience for the pet and the family. This often includes being prepared for many possible scenarios and educating the family as situations change. Even the most challenging cases, when approached with flexibility and compassion, can leave both the family and the practitioner with a sense of peace in the outcome.

REFERENCES

1. Costas R, Karas A, Borns-Weil S. Chill protocol to manage aggressive & fearful dogs. Clinicians Brief 2019;17(5):63–5.
2. Kasten J, Messenger K, Campbell N. Sedative and cardiopulmonary effects of buccally administered detomidine gel and reversal with atipamezole in dogs. Am J Vet Res 2018;79(12):1253–60.
3. VIN. VIN Veterinary drug handbook. Available at: https://www.vin.com/members/cms/project/defaultadv1.aspx?pId=13468&id=7554512. Accessed August 1, 2019.
4. AVMA. AVMA guidelines for the Euthanasia of animals. Available at: https://www.avma.org/KB/Policies/Pages/Euthanasia-Guidelines.aspx. Accessed August 1, 2019.
5. Cooney K. Chapter 3: the appointment in: in-home pet euthanasia techniques. Loveland (CO): Home to Heaven PC; 2011. p. 39–85.
6. Barton L. Respiratory emergencies. Proceedings Atlantic coast veterinary conference 2002. Available at: https://www.vin.com/doc/?id=3845951. Accessed August 1, 2019.
7. Marchitelli B. How exactly does that drug work? Proceedings International Association of Animal Hospice and Palliative Care 2015. Available at: https://www.vin.com/doc/?id=7360510. Accessed August 1, 2019.

Printed and bound by CPI Group (UK) Ltd, Croydon, CR0 4YY

03/10/2024

01040403-0010